Communication Skills in Clinical Practice

Communication Skills in Clinical Practice

(Doctor–Patient Communication)

SECOND EDITION

KR Sethuraman MD PGDHE

Dean, Faculty of Medicine, AIMST University, Malaysia and
Deputy Vice-Chancellor (Academic and International Affairs)
Former Head of Medicine and Medical Education, JIPMER, Puducherry
Email: sethuramankr@hotmail.com

JAYPEE

JAYPEE BROTHERS MEDICAL PUBLISHERS

The Health Sciences Publisher

New Delhi | London

Jaypee Brothers Medical Publishers (P) Ltd

Headquarters
EMCA House
23/23-B, Ansari Road, Daryaganj
New Delhi 110 002, India
Landline: +91-11-23272143, +91-11-23272703
+91-11-23282021, +91-11-23245672
E-mail: jaypee@jaypeebrothers.com

Corporate Office
4838/24, Ansari Road, Daryaganj
New Delhi 110 002, India
Phone: +91-11-43574357
Fax: +91-11-43574314
E-mail: jaypee@jaypeebrothers.com

Overseas Office
J.P. Medical Ltd
83, Victoria Street, London
SW1H 0HW (UK)
Phone: +44 20 3170 8910
E-mail: info@jpmedpub.com

EU GPSR Authorised Representative
Logos Europe, 9 rue Nicolas Poussin
17000, La Rochelle, France
Phone: +33 (0) 6 67 93 73 78
E-mail: contact@logoseurope.eu

Website: www.jaypeebrothers.com
Website: www.jaypeedigital.com

Inquiries for bulk sales may be solicited at: jaypee@jaypeebrothers.com

Communication Skills in Clinical Practice (Doctor-Patient Communication)

First Edition: 2001
Second Edition: 2017
Reprint: **2026**

ISBN 978-93-5152-411-3

Printed in India

DEDICATION

To my wife Anandhi
Behind every author, there is a caretaker
Who fosters freedom to be creative

Preface to the Second Edition

During a clinical career spanning 40 years, a doctor is likely to do around 120,000 to 1,200,000 interviews with patients and their families. Therefore, communication is a core skill which every clinical trainee must learn and cultivate. However, only a few doctors are fortunate to have received some formal training in communication, and even that has proven inadequate in many instances. To remedy the situation there has been a growing emphasis on physician-patient communication in medicine and medical education as evidenced by a plethora of international consensus statements, guidelines for medical schools, and standards for professional practice and education.

During the past decade, since the publication of the first edition of this book, active research in doctor-patient communication has produced provocative and at times conflicting findings: doctors' communications during the medical consultations consist of a mix of instrumental behaviors, which concern their professional expertise in diagnosis and treatment and affective behaviors, which concern doctor-patient relationship. Both these behaviors greatly influence patients' evaluations of the medical care and the outcomes.

Another line of enquiry has shown positive association between facets of doctor-patient communication and medical outcomes, either primary outcomes like reduction in symptoms or of medication, improvement in blood sugar levels, quicker recovery from surgery, and improved health status or secondary outcomes like patient satisfaction, patient empowerment, and patient adherence to therapy.

As the discipline of Doctor-Patient communication matured, the researchers began to recognize the limitations and weaknesses of their studies: most coding systems and empirical approaches to phenomenology are not based on solid theoretical framework; as a result, the research output has resulted in piece-meal findings which are often conflicting. Lack of corroboration among studies is disappointing, and weakens the basis on which scientific knowledge could be constructed.

I have accessed most of the important articles, totalling to above 300, published in the past ten years. The findings of about 70 of the most relevant articles have been incorporated in the second edition to make it current in its scientific content. In view of lack of standardization, several protocols, flow charts and checklists have been published. The more important ones have been cited in full or as usable extracts.

The format of the book has been retained: the first part deals with the core skills of effective communication, the second with the clinical applications and the third goes beyond communication to its raison d'être viz., prudent and patient-centered clinical practice. Practical exercises are suggested at the end of every chapter to enable the readers acquire relevant communication skills by repeated practice.

In 2001, this was the first book on doctor-patient relationship written in South-East Asia. I record my sincere thanks for the support and motivation given by Jaypee Brothers to prepare the second edition of the book. All constructive criticisms are welcome to improve this further.

KR Sethuraman

Preface to the First Edition

One of the things the average doctor does not have time to do is catch up with the things he did not learn in school. If medicine is a mystery to the average man, nearly everything else is a mystery to the average doctor.

—Milton Mayer

The Toronot Consensus of 1991 clearly stated that communication problems in clinical practice are important and common. It also showed that quality of communication is related to health outcome for patients, but that traditional medical education is ineffective at teaching communication. Teaching communication skills should be included at all levels of medical education and, even more importantly, should be a mandatory element of the medical school curriculum and programmes of continuing medical education.

At the Jawaharlal Institute of Postgraduate Medical Education and Research, we have been conducting training on clinical communication skills since 1993 for the students. The materials collected and used by me in these training sessions form the basis of this book. The anecdotes cited are real life incidents culled from my diaries. Anecdotes are perhaps weak as evidences but they are phenomenological observations that convey *what can happen.*

Communication skills are complex. Learning resouces are available from several sources. I have primarily culled learning points on dyadic communication skills from three sources: Clinical, Social exchange and Management perspectives. There are several epistemological differences among the three perspectives, which have been harmonised to some extent to give a holistic view of doctor-patient communication.

This book is aimed at the students, educators and practitioners of clinical medicine and allied sciences, viz. dental, nursing and paramedical disciplines. In this context, the terms "Care-provider" and "Care-seeker" are more appropriate but less elegant than the older terms, Doctor and Patient, which have been retained in this book.

The book has three parts. The first part deals with the core skills of effective communication, the second with clinical applications and the third goes beyond communication to its *raison d'être*, viz. prudent and patient-centred clinical practice. Practical exercises are suggested at the end of every chapter to enable the readers acquire relevant communication skills.

This is perhaps the first book on doctor-patient relationship written in India. All constructive criticisms are welcome to improve this further. Lastly, I record my sincere appreciation of the support given by Jaypee Brothers to medical writers in India, including myself.

KR Sethuraman

Contents

Section 1: Core Skills

Section 2: Clinical Applications

Section 3: Beyond Communication

Annexures

SECTION 1

CORE SKILLS

CHAPTER

1 Doctor–Patient Communication —An Overview

It is a distinct Art to talk Medicine
in the language of non-medical man.

—EH Goodman

Paradoxically, at a time of Internet-based global communication and "Cybermedicine," we are faced with a breakdown in communication between patients and doctors. Increasing patient dissatisfaction, rising numbers of complaints and claims for malpractice and abandonment of conventional medicine for unproven alternatives are the major problems today. In a nation-wide household telephonic survey in US, physicians were *rated lowest on communication skills and on attention to the costs.* A similar survey of physicians showed that they too rated their training the lowest in these same areas. It is apparent that public need for adequate information is not fully met by the doctors.

What do patients want? Most instances of patient dissatisfaction with doctors relate to problems of communication rather than clinical competency. The commonest complaint is, "Doctors do not listen to me." Patients want quality information about their problems and the outlook, more openness about risks of treatment, relief of pain and emotional distress, and professional guidance on what they can do for themselves.

Why is there a communication gap? It is well documented that doctors and patients have different views on what makes good and effective communication; the patients focus on their *life-world* while the doctor, on the *medical-world.* These differences influence the quality of doctor-patient dyad, patient education, compliance and health outcomes.

Why should doctors change? Today, the responsibility for an individual's health care has shifted. Patients today are "health consumers" and want to be active participants in medical decision making. Studies by Kaplan, *et al* have shown that patients tended to leave doctors who failed to involve them in decisions. Many doctors wish to increase their income by increasing their practice load, with a corresponding decrease in time spent per patient. This may backfire if patients abandon the ever-busy and uncaring doctor.

Does quality communication improve health? Studies have documented a correlation between effective communication and improved health outcomes. The outcomes affected were emotional health, resolution of symptoms, pain control, improvement in function, and even in physiological measures such as blood pressure and blood sugar levels (see Hawthorne effect).

Can we learn new communication skills? Firstly, with proper teaching, it is not difficult to acquire communication skills. Secondly, health care is still based on fiduciary relationship that is fostered by sharing of ideas and feelings. Thirdly, effective communication is an interactive process to elicit patient expectations and to counsel them if their expectations are unrealistic.

One should realise that communication is not merely as a set of skills; communicating well is not just a matter of learning discrete pieces of surface behaviour. It is an observable manifestation of appropriate attitude, which may be much more difficult to convey and acquire. It requires development of appropriate attitude as well as cultivation of relevant skills. Appreciating the relevance is the key to self-motivation to learn and change one's behaviour.

UNDERSTANDING COMMUNICATION

Communication is derived from the Latin word *communis*, which means common, or general. That is what we attempt to do when we communicate: we try to find something in common (to share) between the other person(s) and us. Communication is a dynamic, on-going, ever-changing process.

The Process of Communication

Transfer and Sharing of Meanings

Communication involves transfer and sharing of meanings. Meanings may be ideas, images or thoughts expressed in symbols (e.g. writing, speech, music, clothes, smoke, art works, etc.). It is important to realise that messages are not inherent in symbols used. Words, or whatever symbols we use to transmit our messages, have no meanings in themselves. The people involved in the communication process give meaning to these.

Perception

This is another essential component in the process. Perception is defined as *the process of forming impressions about something (a person, an event, or any stimulus that has an effect on our consciousness), and then making a judgement about this.* True communication is not possible without perception. Our perceptions and our judgement are affected/influenced by our senses (i.e. sight, sound, touch, smell and taste).

The Components of Communication

Source/Sender

Source is where a message originates. In a clinical dyad, a doctor and a patient alternate as the source.

Receiver

Receiver refers to a person who receives and interprets a message being transmitted a sender.

Channel

Channel is the means by which a message is transmitted from a source to a receiver. In this case, the means used are interpersonal channels, those involving face-to-face exchange.

Message

Message is the idea that is communicated. The sender selects and organises messages that would be most suited to a particular target audience. The message may be a piece of information, support, encouragement, motivation, correction of errors, or an inquiry into something.

Effects

The purpose of communication is to achieve certain desired results or effects. Effects are changes that occur in a receiver because of transmission of a message. The three main types of effects are:
- Changes in receiver's knowledge
- Changes in receiver's attitude
- Changes in receiver's actions.

Feedback in Communication

Feedback refers to the response or reaction given by the receiver to the sender about his/her ideas and actions. Feedback helps to increase or improve mutual understanding. Both positive and negative feedback should be given when appropriate. Positive feedback is given to encourage or reinforce appropriate ideas or actions. Negative feedback helps to clarify a situation, and make the receiver be aware of how it is perceived by others, reflect on his/her thoughts and actions, and choose to improve or change it.

UNDERSTANDING DOCTOR-PATIENT COMMUNICATION

Since the 70's, attention has shifted from the biomedical side to the humanistic side of medical practice. Eclectic views amalgamate both as a continuous spectrum of biopsychosocial model of medicine (see Table 1.1). Depending on the context, the "Voice of Medicine" has to address the appropriate level in the hierarchy. For instance, talking to a patient about molecular basis of type-1 Diabetes mellitus may be irrelevant if s/he is too poor to buy insulin. Inappropriate focus of the voice of Medicine in an individual case is perhaps the most common cause of communication failure between patients and professionals.

System Analysis of Doctor-Patient Communication

A system has three functional stages of Input, Process and Output/Outcome. A clinical communication can also be conceptualised as a system. Table 1.2 highlights the functional stages of a clinical consultation. It helps one to analyse the communication dyad more

Table 1.1: Hierarchy of biopsychosocial system. The left panel is influenced by social, cultural, economic and environmental factors and the right panel by aetiological factors of genetic and acquired diseases

World	Organ systems
Nation	Organ
Race/Ethnicity	Tissue
Community	Cell
Family	Organelle
Individual	Molecule
	Atom
	Sub-atom

Table 1.2: Clinical dyad as a system

Input variables	*Dyadic process*	*Patient outcome*
Disease characteristics Cultural background Type of patient personality Type of doctor personality Doctor-Patient rapport Doctor behaviour (Control and Affiliation)	Instrumental behaviour - (Problem-solving) Affective behaviour - (Emotional support) Privacy behaviour	*Short term*: Satisfaction, compliance, recall, denial, understanding, arousal of hope, etc. *Long term*: Health status, psychological reaction

meaningfully. (Dyad means 'two similar items' and has been adapted here to indicate the interactions between a doctor-patient pair.)

Doctor Behaviour: Control and Affiliation

Human interpersonal behaviour is universally characterised by 'control behaviour' (to dominate, take charge) and 'affiliation behaviour' (to be friendly and caring, to cooperate with). Research findings consistently reveal that patient satisfaction is positively associated with doctor's affiliation behaviour and negatively associated with doctor's control. Most patients who are satisfied with their medical care have physicians who exhibit high affiliation and low control behaviour with them during consultations.

Components of Dyadic Consultation Process

The interaction in a communication consists of three *component behaviours*:

1. *Instrumental behaviour,* which is task focussed and *cure oriented.* This reflects the patient's need to know, understand and cope with the illness.
2. *Affective behaviour,* which is social and emotional in nature; it is *care oriented.* It reflects the patient's need to feel known and understood as a unique human being (See 'non-person').
3. *Privacy behaviour* in a dyadic analysis refers to the process of exclusion of others from the dyad. Patients—especially females—may feel the need for four types of privacy. They are:
   a. *Physical privacy* concerns the extent to which a patient can control physical accessibility to others, e.g. patients in general wards of teaching hospitals.

b. *Psychological privacy*, refers to the patient's ability to control the interview and influence how much of and to whom personal information is given.
c. *Informational privacy* is to do with confidentiality of patient information, case details and medical records, e.g. psychiatry, surgery, infectious diseases, etc.
d. *Social privacy* refers to control of social contacts in order to maintain status division, e.g. patients from 'high society' tend to avoid interactions with junior doctors and may expect only the senior most professional to attend to them. They may also want an exclusive waiting space to avoid mingling with the commoners.

Patients as Non-Persons

In many clinical settings, the patients are often considered as 'non-persons.'

- Non-persons have no name; they are known by their diseases or bed numbers.
- Non-persons' feelings and opinions do not count. Non-persons are excluded in clinical discussions, even in those that involve risk and treatment preferences. Common examples are bedside discussions on a patient between a surgeon and an anaesthetist, among doctors or between a doctor and a nurse. In fact, if the patient concerned tries to communicate with the professionals, s/he is looked down upon as an 'interfering patient.'
- Non-persons are objects to be dealt with. They do not qualify for 'privacy' (see above). It is all right to intrude into their space—at your convenience—to probe, palpate and do procedures on them. A common example is the de-humanising that is done in most intensive care units.

If you wish to really practise 'patient-centred' medicine, you have to change your mindset and treat the patients as persons (human beings) with individual feelings, ideas and opinions.

Information Needs During a Dyad

Doctors' information needs in a consultation dyad are two:

i. To establish diagnosis.
ii. To plan management.

Patients' needs are also two:

i. To know and understand the origin of symptoms.
ii. To feel known (acceptance of the patient as a 'person' by the doctor) and understood by the doctor (the patient's symptoms taken seriously by the doctor). Feeling known and understood are the missing links in many clinical dyads.

Approach to Doctor–Patient Dyad

Physician centred approach is one in which the doctor leads the consultation dyad in explaining the disease and its treatment ("voice of Medicine"). *Patient centred approach* is one in which the patient leads the consultation dyad concerning the areas of his/her expertise viz., symptoms, disability, treatment preferences and concerns regarding illness ("voice of Lifeworld"). The latter approach needs appropriate physician responses, which enables patients to express all their reasons ("agendas") for consulting the doctor, including their symptoms, thoughts, feelings and expectations. An ideal medical interview combines both approaches.

Attributes of Effective Communication ("Voice of Medicine")

i. *Accuracy*: Valid content presented accurately.
ii. *Availability*: The message is available to the end user at the time of its need.
iii. *Timeliness*: The message is conveyed when the audience is in need of and most receptive to it.
iv. *Understandable*: Follows the norms of clarity, choice of words appropriate for the patient.
v. *Culturally competent*: The message, the medium and the mode of delivery are appropriate for the culture of the target group.
vi. *Reliability*: The patient feels s/he can rely on the source, and the message.
vii. *Evidence based*: The message as well as the communication method is evidence based.
viii. *Balance*: Presentation is balanced, e.g., felt need vs. real need, benefit and risk, cost and benefit, natural history and outlook after intervention, etc.
ix. *Consistency*: The message is internally consistent over time and externally consistent with other sources of unbiased information.
x. *Repetition*: Repeated delivery to reinforce the message.

Factors Influencing a Consultation Dyad

One should realise that in addition to the professional mediated attributes listed above, other factors influence the process and outcome of a consultation dyad. Major factors are—

i. Patient attributes like personality, literacy and socio-cultural placement, etc.
ii. Professional attributes like personality (friendly, unfriendly) and concern (concerned, not concerned).
iii. Doctor-patient relationship (clinical, therapeutic, personal or intimate).
iv. Severity and type of disease.
v. Patient expectation and agenda.
vi. Type of treatment (invasive or not, level of risky, cost, etc.)
vii. Time available for dyad.

Categories of Doctor–Patient Misunderstanding

Misunderstanding leads to most of the litigation. Awareness of common reasons for doctor-patient misunderstanding may help one to nip the problem in the bud.

- Patient information unknown to doctor.
- Doctor information unknown to patient.
- Conflicting information given (verbal/non-verbal mismatch; doctor to doctor variations)
- Disagreement about attribution of causation or nature of illness (knowledge gap).
- Failure of communication about doctor's decision.
- Relationship factors (Dysfunctional dyad).

Language in Consultation Dyads

Doctors are bilingual; they use medical language (ML) that is technically correct and, everyday language (EL) that is easily understood by patients. Experienced doctors often switch between ML and EL in order to communicate better with their patients.

Patients may also try to use ML rather than EL. Quite often this leads to confusion. Studies have shown that a majority (64%) of patients misunderstands common health terms. 'Allergy' for a lay person in India often means things s/he detests or finds unsuitable for any reason. 'Tension' is similarly used for any kind of stress, anger or irritation. 'Gastric' or 'gas' may mean eructation, indigestion, flatulence, reflux, etc. So it is prudent for a doctor to verify what exactly the patient means whenever s/he uses medical terms.

Closure of Consultation Dyads

Physicians need to improve their communication skills in the closing phase of the medical interview. In a study by White, *et al*, the communication between physicians and patients in the closing phase of the dyad was analysed. The physicians initiated the closing in 86% of the visits. They clarified the plan of care in 75% of the visits. They asked whether the patients had more questions only in 25% of the cases. New problems during closure were associated with less information exchange between physicians and patients, fewer orientation statements by physicians and long closures (> 2 minutes). In 21% of the cases, the patients raised new problems at the end of the consultation. Orienting the patients to the flow of the consultation, assessing their beliefs, checking for understanding, and addressing psychosocial issues early on may decrease the number of new problems introduced by them in the final moments of the visit.

Patient Outcome in a Consultation Dyad

Outcome is defined as an observable consequence that occurs after a consultation dyad—or a part of the dyad—is completed. There are several components of patient outcome: Knowledge and understanding of the illness, coping with illness, quality of life, psychological reaction like anxiety and depression, satisfaction, compliance, recovery, sick-role, and social support, etc.

Physician behaviour, if supportive, may result in reinforcing the patient's self-confidence, motivation and a positive view of health resulting in a feeling of medico-social support. Such patients may even consult the same physician repeatedly for social support rather than medical treatment. A doctor who is unaware of this may wonder why such patients bother them repeatedly with minor ailments. Experienced physicians have a collection of 'elderly well,' who consult them every now and then for social support and soothe-saying rather than medical treatment (see 'Hawthorne effect').

Patients 'Ranking of Doctors' Communication Behaviours

I like my doctor to

- explain the reasons for my treatment
- listen to me when I speak
- talk to me in simple language
- encourage me to ask questions
- give me information without me asking for it
- ask me what my emotional feelings are about my illness or treatment
- maintain eye-contact when either they or I are talking
- seek my point of view about my illness or treatment
- smile when communicating with me

I may like my doctor to be
- serious when communicating with me.

I do not like my doctor to
- discuss only medical matters with me
- wait until I ask before informing me about my illness or treatment.

Good Doctor–Patient Relationship

Being multi-facetted and multi-dimensional, doctor-patient relationship is one of the most complex social relationships. It is difficult to define this complex relationship.
According to many studies, the necessary ingredients for *goodness* are:

- Mutual trust
- Honesty, and devotion to patient-care.
- Social orientation
- Non-judgmental attitude
- Friendliness and empathy
- Conveying interest and a desire to help
- Giving patients compliments
- Making inoffensive personal remarks, laughing or making jokes.

Carl Rogers' client-centred model comprising of *empathy, respect, warmth, genuineness and unconditional acceptance* also indicates components of good doctor-patient relationship.

Concept of Empathy

Empathy is "feeling with" the patient, while sympathy is "feeling for" the patient. Empathy is a *cerebral* response, while sympathy is a *visceral* response.
Empathic relationship consists of:

- Eliciting patient's feelings
- Paraphrasing and reflecting on what the patient has said
- Using silent pauses appropriately (for reflection and introspection)
- Listening to what the patient says and also what s/he is trying to say or is unable to say (to read *between lines* and *beyond lines*)
- Encouragement
- Non-verbal behaviour that complements the above.

SUMMARY

"A strong, therapeutic, and effective relationship is the sine qua non of physician-patient communication". A patient-centered or relationship-centered approach to care emphasizes both the patient's disease and his or her illness experience. This requires eliciting the patient's story of illness while guiding the interview through a process of diagnostic reasoning. This approach regards the physician-patient relationship as a partnership, and respects patients' active participation in decision making. The ideas, feelings, and values of both the patient and the physician influence the relationship." (The Kalamazoo Consensus Statement). This chapter is meant as an overview of the doctor-patient communication process. The details of different aspects of the doctor-patient communication process follow in the subsequent chapters.

BIBLIOGRAPHY

1. Donald J Kiesler, Stephen M Auerbach. Integrating measurement of control and affiliation in studies of physician-patient interaction: The interpersonal circumplex. Social Science & Medicine 2003;57: 1707-22.
2. Francis PHN, et al. Gaps in doctor-patient communication. NEJM 1969;280:535-40.
3. Kaplan SH, Greenfield S, Gandek B, Rogers WH, Ware JE. Characteristics of physicians with participatory decision-making styles. Ann Intern Med 1996;124:497-504.
4. LML Ong, et al. Doctor-patient communication: A Review of Literature. Social Science & Medicine 1995;40:903-18.
5. Leckie J, Bull R, Vrij A. The development of a scale to discover outpatients' perceptions of the relative desirability of different elements of doctors' communication behaviours. Patient Education and Counseling 2006;64: 69-77.
6. McBride CA, Shugars DA, DiMatteo MR, Lepper HS, O'Neil EH, Damush TM. The physician's role. Views of the public and the profession on seven aspects of patient care. Archives of Family Medicine. 1994;3(11):948-53.
7. Siegfried Meryn, Improving doctor-patient communication. Not an option, but a necessity (Editorial) BMJ 1998;316:1922-30.
8. The Kalamazoo Consensus Statement—Essential Elements of Communication in Medical Encounters. Acad. Med. 2001;76:390-393. Available at http://journals.lww.com/academicmedicine/toc/2001/04000 (accessed on 18-09-2010) (*vide* Annexe - 3).
9. White J, Levinson W, Roter D. "Oh, by the way...": The closing moments of the medical visit. Journal of General Internal Medicine. 1994;(1):24-8.

EXERCISES

Group Discussion Following Video-triggers

Video-triggers from movies like "Anand" (Hindi), "The Citadel", "Patch Adams", etc. or from the plethora of medical TV-serials like ER, Mercy, Dr House, Grey's Anatomy, etc., highlighting various aspects of doctor-patient consultation dyad have to be collected. Each trigger, not more than 1 to 5 minutes long, will be followed by group discussion on its message.

Case Studies on Lifeworld

Using the multi-dimensional model of health care as a guide, each pair of students will talk with an in-patient to identify various social, cultural, environmental and economic factors that influence health-seeking behaviour in each instance (See Annexure 2 for the model).

Practice Sessions

Students practise consultation skills with real or simulated patients. Repeated practise is needed to assess improvement over time. Their proficiency can be rated using 'Communication Assessment Tool' (CAT), which is tested to be a reliable and valid instrument for measuring patient perceptions of physician's interpersonal and communication skills.*

*Ref: Makoul G, Krupat E, Chang C. Measuring patient views of physician communication skills: Development and testing of the Communication Assessment Tool. Patient Education and Counseling 2007;67:333-42.

The real or simulated patient has to fill up the brackets with his/her rating of the doctor's performance.

Using a five-point scale: 1 = poor, 2 = fair, 3 = good, 4 = very good, 5 = excellent

The Doctor

1. Greeted me in a way that made me feel comfortable [ ]
2. Treated me with respect [ ]
3. Showed interest in my ideas about my health [ ]
4. Understood my main health concerns [ ]
5. Paid attention to me (looked at me, listened) [ ]
6. Let me talk without interruptions [ ]
7. Gave me as much information as I wanted [ ]
8. Talked in terms I could understand [ ]
9. Checked to be sure I understood everything [ ]
10. Encouraged me to ask questions [ ]
11. Involved me in decisions as much as I wanted [ ]
12. Discussed the next steps [ ]
13. Showed care and concern [ ]
14. Spent the right amount of time with me [ ]

(*The rating can be simplified as a three-point rating scale: 0 = not at all, 1 = did to some extent, 2 = did to my satisfaction. CAT focuses on the achievement of communication tasks rather than specific ways of accomplishing them. It is a practical, simple and straight forward tool that is understandable by patients across literacy levels.*)

CHAPTER

2

Questioning Skills

I keep six honest serving men (they taught me all I know):
Their names are What and Why and When
And How and Where and Who.

—R Kipling in "*The serving men*"

INTRODUCTION

Questions elicit patients' perceptions, opinions, feelings and understanding. These are of great importance in the practice of *patient centred management*. Questioning skills are not difficult for a doctor to acquire. Questioning must be followed by active listening to the patient. However, far too many doctors do most of the talking, while their patients sit back, patiently trying to listen and hope to see the light.

Uses of Questions

- *Fixing initial appointment*: This avoids time wastage for both parties, for example, in redirecting a patient with a seizure to a neurologist instead of a cardiologist as desired by the patient.
- *Initial case assessment* by history and physical examination.
- *Qualifying and prioritising* patient's problems.
- *Discussing* the cost-benefit and risk-benefit of the options.
- *Assessing* family support, financial status and spending capacity to initiate and sustain treatment till its completion.
- *Considering various management options* and deciding on the most suitable option for the patient.
- *Handling concerns*, doubts, misunderstanding, and unrealistic expectation.
- *Pacing your presentation to patients*: A common error is to rush through your presentation. After all, you have delivered similar messages to many patients in many different settings.

Therefore, after a while, it seems like old news to you. However, it may be new and strange to your patient.

- *Buying time*: It is common during consultations to come across a patient who asks very complex questions that challenge the limits of your knowledge. While the patient deserves an answer, you also need some time to think before you give it. The best way to buy time is to respond to the question with a question of your own.
- *Negotiating* terms and conditions of any interventional procedures for diagnosis or treatment.
- *Guiding them in the correct direction*: If you know the direction in which your patients need to think, you should be able to get them there through a series of questions. Every time a patient says yes or makes a choice, s/he has increased his/her commitment to accept your advice. For example: "Don't you want to get rid of the excess fat?" (Yes, I do.) " Do you want to try non-surgical option first?" (Yes, I do.) "Would you prefer an inexpensive remedy?" (Yes, I do.) etc.
- *Assessing compliance* and adherence to therapy.

BENEFITS OF EFFECTIVE QUESTIONING

Effective Questioning

i. Often yields vital information, the importance of which may escape the patient until pointed out
ii. Helps to control the consultation process efficiently
iii. Helps to build rapport and develop trust
iv. Helps to minimise misunderstanding
v. Helps to reduce patient resistance to accept treatment advice and improve compliance.

Obtain Vital Information

"A prudent question is one-half of wisdom"—Francis Bacon.

"What you do not know can not hurt you" and "Ignorance is bliss" can be deadly concepts in doctor-patient dyads. Knowledge is power—power to manage the case more prudently and efficiently. Understanding the socio-economic status, personal motives, needs, goals and problems of patients will help in planning holistic and effective case management.

Do not assume. Do not presume. Elicit reliable information from the patients. Astute assumptions that you can meet the patient's needs and solve the problems may often prove wrong. A well-dressed middle class patient may appear rich but may complain about the cost of therapy and drop out. On the other hand, a poorly dressed illiterate villager may have hectares of land and may be willing to pay for the best treatment. So never attempt to advise on management options until you have completely determined the various factors that influence the plan of case management.

Control the Dyad Sans Offence

Control does not mean aggressively setting the agenda and dominating the interview all the time. Achieve control and lead the direction of the dyad by:

- Intervening as and when required with comments and by seeking clarifications, and
- Asking pertinent questions to patients who digress to bring them back on track.

While questioning, appear considerate, low-key, alert and not pushy. Show empathy. Do not pressurise the patient and do not appear to be coercive or manipulative.

Build Rapport and Trust

Do not shoot questions like a charging bull focussed on nothing but the patient's medical problems. It converts the dyad into an interrogation. Except when giving management advice, you should talk less than 50% of the time. *Patient-centredness* means making her/him feel like the "co-provider" of health care and not like a passive recipient. An old saying makes this point well: *"If they do not share, they would not care."*

Finding out the felt needs of a patient does not mean giving in or losing control. It only reveals your sensitivity to the patient's perspective of things (voice of the lifeworld). For example, a young woman with type-1 diabetes mellitus may feel that her diabetes should be controlled without any insulin injections. Unless we find out why she feels that way, we may not be able to convince her of the need to comply with insulin therapy (see *probing questions*).

Minimise Misunderstanding

Patients misunderstand their doctors quite often. This leads to frustration, hurt feelings, loss of trust, anger and even litigation. Do not 'smooth over' a patients doubts and anxieties. Develop the fine art of conveying *realistic optimism*. The best way to ensure that a person has understood whatever you have said is to ask him to repeat it in his own words (feedback).

Promote Compliance

All patients have questions, concerns, reservations, objections or fear regarding health care services. Unless you can elicit these and adequately address these, you can not improve patient compliance.

Many patients may play along with you initially and the treatment plan may seem to be proceeding smoothly. At the point of no return, when they have to comply with "the doctor's orders", these patients will drop out. Fearing ridicule or castigation, many of them will not even inform you why they have dropped off the treatment at its crucial point (see *deceptive patient*).

If you wish to avoid the frustration of dealing with such deceptive games by your patients, do these:

- Elicit patients' fears and concerns regarding health care options
- Listen non-judgementally and allow your patients to freely express their fears and concerns
- Try to identify the likely points of patient resistance.

THREE DIMENSIONS OF A QUESTION

Medical students are repeatedly told never to ask leading questions to patients. There is hardly any discussion on different dimensions of a question and the place for each one of them in a doctor-patient dyad. The net result is that the students totally avoid asking leading questions, at times missing vital information. They also ask complex questions mixing two or three queries in a single sentence.

There are three dimensions to a question:

i. Open-ended or closed-ended
ii. Direct or indirect
iii. Leading or non-leading.

Let us now study these dimensions and their value in a medical interview.

Open-ended Question

An open-ended question (OEQ) does not restrict the response but permits wide ranging answers. Such questions are best used at the beginning of a dyad. "Tell me about your health problems" is a common example of OEQ used to open a medical interview.
Use of such OEQs at the beginning of an interview helps to:

- Get the patient "open out" and to help him/her to "start talking"
- Begin a productive interview
- Establish rapport with the patient as OEQs make him/her feel important, intelligent, respected and seemingly in charge of the dyad.

The key words of OEQs are *what, why and how*. Some examples: "How is your pain today?" "Why do you think it is related to what you ate?" "What is your major concern now?" Try to develop skills of asking OEQs—using what, why and how—during the initial part of an interview and at least 50% of the time thereafter.

OEQs have their drawbacks too. A patient with multiple problems may go off on a tangent. Novice medicos often enquire about 'any problems?' and get a detailed reply on the financial problems currently troubling the patient; also, a verbose patient may talk at length to describe a minor symptom. The solution is not to stop asking OEQs but to take control and bring the patient back on track by summarising or asking another question.

At times, patients with a major life-event in the past, link it up with the current problem. A common scene in our female outpatient wing is a tubectomised patient relating her 3-day fever to the tubectomy done several years earlier! If such life events dominate a patient's initial concern, it is good to allow them to voice it briefly. One should not rebuke them for linking up unconnected events. Any clarification in this regard is best done, at the time of closure of the dyad. For example, I often use the Tamil saying, "W*hat is the connection between a bald-head and the knee-cap?"* to give them insight and to elicit a smile but I say it only after solving the present problem of the patient.

Closed-ended Question

A closed-ended question (CEQ) permits only a limited (yes/no) type of responses. CEQs should be limited to specific areas that require short and specific answers. It is an excellent tool to clarify some point, for example, "...did you say gripping pain?" The key words of CEQ are *when, where and who.* Some examples: "When did you get these symptoms?", "Where does it hurt?" and "Who treated you earlier?" Some other phrases for CEQ are, 'Am I ...', 'Would you ...', 'Can it ...', etc.

CEQ, if used too much, may make the patient feel restricted, subservient, manipulated and even angry. The interview will have rough and abrupt quality and may cause patient dissatisfaction. To get a feel of this, just ask your colleague to ask you a set of ten CEQs in a rapid sequence. The difference between grilling and interviewing will then be obvious.

Closed-ended questioning is best used to supplement an OEQ to clarify the patient's views or to confirm your impressions. They are also of use in eliciting routine information like name, age, address, etc.

Direct Question

A direct question (DQ) gets right to the point. It is efficient. It is a straightforward, clear and no-nonsense type of eliciting answers. It can be open-ended ('what happened?') or closed-ended ('who knocked you down?').

The main drawback of DQ is that it is abrupt and may put-off new patients who do not trust you yet. If you wish to elicit useful information, it is better to limit DQs when dealing with new cases. Stronger the rapport, more direct can be your questioning style. Many of us use this approach instinctively. Direct questioning may appear tactless and rude when exploring sensitive areas like addictions and sexual habits.

Indirect Question

An indirect question (IDQ) elicits answer in an oblique and roundabout manner. It is gentle and non-threatening. In a suspected case of battered wife syndrome, a DQ like, "Does your husband beat you?' is likely to fail, while indirect questions on her married life may yield clues, especially through her non-verbal behaviour (body-language). IDQ also helps to save your face when straying into such off-limit areas. You can retract by saying, "If you do not want talk about it now, it is okay with me."

IDQ is the questioning mode of choice when eliciting sensitive information from patients in high positions, of those with high self-esteem (priests, teachers, village headman, etc.). While probing sensitive areas by IDQs, you may use one of the four techniques described below.

The "If We Knew" Technique

An example: "*If we know* that you have perhaps given some anti-diarrhoea medicine to your child, then I could surmise why she has bloated abdomen and is so drowsy."

This approach may work when the parents of a child with diarrhoea seem unduly reluctant to talk about the medications given to her. By focussing on how the information would help in better managing the case, you may coax them to come out with the fact that they have give opioid drug to stop the diarrhoea. The 'If we knew' approach looks ahead and focuses on what is to be done. In contrast, direct questioning may only promote feelings of guilt and remorse without helping you solve the problems at hand.

The Reference Base Technique

An example: "This drug therapy costs Rs. 5,000 per month. Is it all right for you? Can you manage to take the treatment for a full year?"

In this technique, the physician gives an estimate as a reference point for further discussions before taking a final decision. You can even soften this some more by saying, "Usually this costs Rs. 5000 per month and many patients do say that it is too expensive. I wonder if you also have any such reservation." By indicating that it is all right to feel hesitant, you coax them to come out with their true feelings.

The Rough Estimate Technique

Use this technique when you want a reference point from the patient to start further discussions. Ask for a vague answer within a reasonable range. To a physical instructor, who is reluctant to discuss how many cigarettes he smokes, you may say, "Many active persons do smoke. What would be your consumption? About 20 packs, 50 packs or 100 packs per month?" It is a prudent habit to overstate such estimates of bottles of liquor consumed or packs of cigarettes smoked so that the patient does not mind accepting a figure far less than the suggested figure.

The Third Person Technique

This technique is reserved for the reticent patient who is not forthcoming despite gentle IDQ by the earlier methods. Here, you talk about a hypothetical "third person" that has similar problems like the present case and ask his/her opinion as to what could be done. This exposes the "hot buttons" of the patient without offence. The patient can also agree or disagree with what happened to the 'third person' without seeming to offend you.

However, the hypothetical third person is coloured by your personal bias; therefore, this ploy may not elicit true responses from the patient. You may end up realising that the person in front of you is far different from the imaginary 'third person'. (I have never used this technique due to this limitation.) However, a few patients may use this technique to get your opinion on their problems, which is too sensitive or private to be shared with you.

Leading Question

A leading question (LQ) is carefully phrased and designed to influence a patient in the manner implied by the question. LQs may induce the patient to 'play along' to avoid the embarrassment of further discussions on a sensitive topic and to avoid loss of respect. Thus, LQs can distort patient history and subjective elements of physical examination. Therefore, LQs have been almost banished from the repertoire of a clinician.

However, LQs do have an important role in *clarifying* or *confirming* and in *counselling* patients (the 3-Cs of medical interview). Some examples:

- "Do not you mean that despite the illness, you still want to continue smoking?" is an LQ that confirms what the patient just said.
- "Do not you realise that smoking may make the treatment ineffective?" clarifies if the patient has understood the risks.
- "Is not it true that you love your family and would like to live a long healthy life?" is an LQ that leads to counselling.

The key words of LQs are "do not you..." "is not it true..." "can not we...", etc. These work well in the 3-Cs of an interview if the following tactics are adopted:

- Always phrase LQs in a neutral, non-intimidating way. For example, in a patient with fever for three weeks, asking, "How many doctors have you consulted before coming to me?" may not elicit the truth, as the public generally believes that doctors get upset if you tell them about any earlier treatment. A more tactful LQ like, "Your fever is three weeks old. How have you taken treatment till now?" is more likely to reveal the truth.
- Always ask LQs in a friendly, open conversational way.
- The patient should be able to respond freely and openly without feeling coerced.
- While asking a set of LQs, vary the key phrases.

To sum up, when used judiciously, leading questions enhance the quality of an interview, especially in the 3-Cs of clarifying, confirming and counselling.

Non-leading Question

A non-leading question (NLQ) is phrased in a neutral and unbiased way so that the patient does not feel pressurised or obliged to give the answer you may be looking for. A good NLQ may make the patient wonder what you are looking for, as the question gives no clues as to the expected answer.

"*Why do you want to kill yourself? Do not you want to stop drinking?*" is an offensive form of LQ. "*Would you rather not give up drinking?*" is a gentle form of LQ. "*What do you intend to do about your drinking habit?*" is non-leading and he is free to give a wide ranging response.

Three-dimensional Analysis

Any question can be analysed as an open or closed, direct or indirect and leading or non-leading type. "*What is your name?*" is open, direct and non-leading; "*Do you smoke?*" is closed, direct and non-leading. Classifying and coding questions this way (O/C - D/I - L/N) helps one to quickly master the technique of intuitively asking the most appropriate question in a given situation.

EFFECTIVE QUESTIONING SKILLS

The function of genius is not to give new answers, but to pose new questions—which time and mediocrity can solve.

—Hugh Trevor-Roper

The objective of questioning is to elicit maximum information relevant to the case in the shortest possible time using purposeful, probing and inoffensive questions. The following are some tips on effective questioning.

1. Explain the purpose of the question; explain how answering it will be of use to the patient.
2. Begin with friendly questions and then ask relevant ones.
3. Ask easy, clearly worded questions in a simple way. Ask one question at a time. Do not ask mixed (two or more) or complex (double negative) questions.
4. To get the patient to 'open up', ask for her/his *feelings* and not merely *thoughts*. For example, instead of "Do not you *think* that the operation is essential?" ask, "What do you *feel* about the proposed operation?"
5. Probe in a general way about the patient's problems, needs, and lifestyle, and prioritise the major problems. Then probe deeply into areas of concern. This is like using a torch beam—the broad beam of soft light picks up objects of concern which are then observed under the bright central beam of light. Torch beam model is as efficient as it is effective in eliciting information. *Caution*: While this approach is useful in chronic problems, the initial general probe wastes time in acute emergencies. It is prudent to 'get on with it' in such instances.
6. Use patient's name wherever possible. It makes rapport building easier. *Caution*: In India and the Orient, it is impolite to call out the names of the elderly, the leaders and married

women. You may address them by their initials as done in the South, or call them "seniors" in the local dialect. Later, you can even give them a friendly nickname.

7. Do not ask too many closed-ended questions (rapid-fire type) and convert the dyad into a grilling session. To busy residents, this method seems very fast and efficient but the information collected this way will have several errors and in the end, prove imprudent.
8. Wait until the previous question is fully answered before moving on to the next. The time gap between the end of a question and the beginning of the answer is termed *response latency*, which is normally about half a second. Excited persons may take only 0.3 sec to respond while depressed patients may take several seconds to respond.
9. If the answer to a question is important, ensure that the patient has answered satisfactorily before moving on. For example, a stoic person may not give clear-cut answers to questions on anginal syndrome. It is our job to ensure that he has given us the complete picture.
10. Do not make a habit of rhetoric questioning. A patient may wonder, "Why is he asking me all this if he is going to answer all of them?"
11. Avoid *flashy* questions like, "It is great to be treated by me, do not you think so?" and *stupid* questions (with obvious answers) like, "You want to control your sugar, do not you?"
12. Stay away from *nosy* questions that are too personal, sensitive or confidential. If they are important, convince the patient first and then ask in the indirect mode.
13. Avoid questions that turn the patients off and those that make them feel guilty, stupid, wrong, inferior or angry. An example: "Do you honestly believe that you can omit the medicines and live happily ever after?" At times, these may be used in non-compliant patients with whom you have a good rapport when other methods of counselling fail to make them see reason.
14. Show confidence when asking questions, especially on personal details, addictions, sexual habits, etc. Maintain a comfortable eye contact after the question.
15. Plan your questioning strategy and tactics before you see chronic cases on follow-up.
16. Be proactive. Anticipate all possible reactions from a patient (crying, shame, anger, etc.) and be ready with your next move. For example, when discussing the need for surgery, the patient response may vary from total acceptance to total rejections with all gradations in between. You should plan tactics of handling any of them.

ADVANCED QUESTIONING SKILLS

Once you gain confidence in asking questions in different ways as mentioned above, you can go on to contextual, patient-centred questioning mode. The predominant styles useful in doctor-patient dyads are described below.

Basic Qualifying Questions

You may wonder why anyone would want to give advice without first assessing the listener's needs and motive. Yet, most doctors launch right into therapeutic advice before confirming that they have a receptive patient. Basic qualifying questions (BQQ) help in assessing the needs, motive and readiness of a patient. BQQs have to be asked at different times during a consultation to ensure that the patient is receptive and likely to comply with your advice (see '4+ yes' and 'deceptive patient').

Initial Contact

The easiest way of asking initial BQQs is to enquire: (i) why the patient has chosen to consult you and (ii) why at that particular time.

Assessing the Patient's Initial Receptivity

When you want to ask a patient about undergoing an elective surgery but feel that it is too soon to ask such a strong question, you can soften the question and still assess the patient's readiness. An example: "Ms J, suppose we were to discover a non-functioning gallbladder filled with stones, what would you do?" If she says she would probably get it removed, continue with your presentation on risks and benefits of surgery.

The Rephrased BQQ

Rephrase the BQQ in situations where the prospect does not give you a definite "yes" commitment to your BQQ, but responds instead with a "maybe" or "perhaps." To a patient who is hesitant to say yes to an elective cholecystectomy, rephrase the BQQ and ask again: "Ms J, shall we discuss the need for surgery again after the ultrasound report is available?"

The Customised BQQ

One of the most effective ways to ask a BQQ is to listen very carefully to your patient for his or her explicit needs. The patient will reveal them as you ask your information-gathering questions. As you learn the specific needs, build your BQQ around them. To a patient who does not want any therapy due to aversion to injections, you may ask, "If I can prescribe something taken by mouth, which is as effective as an injection, will you take it?"

The Combined BQQ

This is actually a combination of a soft BQQ and a strong BQQ:

"Suppose our hospital can address your problems to your total satisfaction, will you really be ready to get started with this line of treatment?" This is useful in coaxing 'fence-sitters' to make up their mind.

The Indirect (Camouflaged) BQQ

Sometimes when you are dealing with high-level professionals, especially health professionals, you may want to ask the BQQ a little differently, so that it does not sound rude. Here is an example: "Maybe we can help you; maybe we can not. You have to decide that. But if you are convinced that we can be of help, when do you see yourself getting started on therapy?"

Probing Questions

Although probing questions are harder to ask, they are effective in eliciting information which a patient may not feel is important. Your goal in asking probing questions is to help the patient to think. Because that person may have forgotten all of the problems involved, or is not aware of all of them, probing questions usually uncover additional and related problems.

Ideally, you should take *implied problems* and convert them into *explicit problems* to help the prospect gain insight into the nature of his/her illness and its management. Ask questions such as:

- "*What effect does this ...(illness) have on you?*" (Your life-style, morale, quality of life, etc.)—An open and direct Q.
- "*Does not this cause problems in your...?*"—A closed and leading Q.
- "*I sense you are frightened by... Am I right?*"
- "*Do you also worry about . . .?*"
- "*Can you think back and see if the episodes of seizure have any relationship with lack of sleep or mental tension?*"

One of the benefits of asking probing questions is that you do not do much of the talking. As you listen for problems and probe deeper and deeper, the patient will begin gain insight and will look to you for some helpful advice. Then, the two of you can explore solutions together. For example, most of my patients with angina realise its relationship with mental stress and eating a heavy meal only when I probe deeply into their symptoms. This insight renders therapeutic advice easy to accept and follow.

Problem-exploring Questions

This is a type of probing question focussing on "soft hints" from a patient, usually by way of non-verbal behaviour or picked up by reading between the lines. The goal of problem implication questions is to help patients identify their "implied" needs. For example, an elderly couple with good control of their diabetes may show body language of concern/fear while one of them says, "Thanks to you, the diabetes is under good control even though we are a little pre-occupied with other things."

If you catch the hint, you may begin your questions in the following ways:

- "You said you had other concerns. What did you mean by that?"
- "Would you explain about the *other things* that preoccupy you both?"
- "As your doctor, what should I know about these other things that seem to worry you both?"

Solution-exploring Questions

If problem-exploring questions are "unhappy" probing questions, solution-exploring questions are just the reverse. These get the patient to talk on possible solutions to the problems discussed earlier. Ask hypothetical questions such as:

"If we could solve that problem, what would that do in terms of your ... (employment, hobbies, income, sex-life, etc.)?"

"Would not that ... (treatment) also give you more freedom to do the things you like doing?"

"What other benefits are obvious to you if we can help you to control your ... (BP, sugar level, fits, etc.)?"

Multi-layered Probing Question (MLPQ)

Multi-layered Probing Question (MLPQ) is a complex question consisting of three parts. It is useful in initiating and sustaining an in-depth discussion. An MLPQ permits one to question a patient in the "evidence based mode."

The three parts of MLPQs are:

- Statement of fact or evidence
- Observation (optional)
- Probing question

MLPQs are quite effective in talking to health professionals who come as patients for consultations. Lay public is often confused by complex MLPQs; therefore, avoid asking such questions to them.

The Statement of Fact

The statement of fact (or evidence) is critical because it allows you to lure the patient into an in-depth dialogue. Address an important issue that concerns your patient. Depending on the circumstances, this issue might be innovative therapy, new technology, safety, cost-benefit ratio, risk-benefit ratio or efficiency. Previous experience with a patient often helps one to decide what would be his/her important concerns.

Four prerequisites for stating facts are:

1. Facts must address an issue of concern for the patient.
2. Facts should be incontrovertible.
3. Facts must come from a credible source.
4. Refrain from mentioning your own opinions.

The Observation (Opinion)

This element can play a dual role in your questioning technique. It can help support your statement of fact by lending credibility ("Most experts also feel that way"). It can also give a contrary perspective that can provoke an alternate point of view ("Our Journal said this, but the Review said that"). In either case, you can use this element to your advantage by either strengthening your viewpoint or contradicting the fact under discussion. This technique can lead your patient in either direction and still help build your rapport.

This step is optional, so use it only if it makes sense to do so. For example, this is a good technique to use to push a vacillating patient (a *fence-sitter*) off the fence.

The Probing Question

This part asks the patient about his/her views and says how it compares with what you discussed in the earlier "fact" stage. The probing questions must be in *open mode*, i.e, should not include a closed-ended option at the end (e.g. "do not you agree?"), because you will force the patient to a 'yes' or 'no' answer.

For example, to a nurse who is a long-term diabetic, one may ask an open-ended MLPQ like this one: "Recent studies stress the need to improve glycaemic control. This is supported by several leading diabetologists. Tell me your experience in monitoring your own therapy. How does it compare with current standards?"

Value of Probing Questions

i. They uncover the implied needs and converted them into explicit needs
ii. They help the patient to think about the consequences of not solving the problems

iii. If you probe and then just listened quietly, they coax the patients to confide in you, their frustrations, concerns, needs and motivations
iv. They are likely to be effective in *enabling the patients* to gain insight and cope with their illness-related problems.

SUMMARY

Learning how and when to ask open/closed, direct/indirect and leading/non-leading questions can hone the skills of effective questioning during a doctor patient dyad. Later, advanced skills can be acquired by the use of basic qualifying questions that assess patients' needs and readiness to accept therapeutic advice. Probing questions that focus on exploring problems and solutions are of use in in-depth interviewing. Multi-layered probing question is the most complex of these and needs to be selectively used with knowledgeable patients who like evidence based interviews.

BIBLIOGRAPHY

1. Articles on "Questioning Skills" in www.mindtools.com.
2. Slesinski RA. Effective Questioning. In *How to Skyrocket Your Sales.*, UBSPD, N.Delhi, 1995.
3. Wozny DA and Watson JC. Counselors' Questioning Skills Repertoire: What We Use and What We Don't. Available at www.counseling.org/Resources/Library/VISTAS/vistas06/vistas06.30.pdf (accessed on 18-09-2010).

PRACTICAL EXERCISES

1. *Coding Questions*: Students pair off. One asks any clinical question that comes to his/her mind. The partner classifies and codes each question in the 3-dimensions (O/C; D/I; L/NL). Then the pair switches roles. At the end, the tutor can arrange a plenary session where each pair will present samples of each type of questions or offer examples to the type indicated by the tutor.
2. *Converting Questions*: Students pair off. One asks a type of question to the other who has to convert it to the other type, i.e. open to closed, direct to indirect or leading to non-leading question. In the first round, only one dimension is converted. Later on, the students can attempt to convert two dimensions in each of the questions, e.g., open and indirect to closed and direct. The students who are very adept at this may be given the last tough round of converting all 3-dimensions, e.g. a closed, direct and leading question is converted to an open, indirect and non-leading type.
3. *Simulated Interview*: Students pair off. One acts as a patient and the other as a doctor. A situation, which requires indirect questioning, is simulated. The 'doctor-student' then asks in one of the four modes of indirect questioning, e.g. "if we knew..." technique. The 'patient-student' keeps track of slips and mistakes committed by the 'doctor.' The tutor conducts a plenary session, where these interviews are discussed and doubts clarified.
4. *Advanced Skills Practice (For Postgraduates)*: Simulated doctor-patient dyads can be arranged and situations contrived so that basic qualifying questions (BQQ) and probing questions can be practised. Simulated patients who need elective surgical procedures are good examples to practise BQQ. Seizure, angina, peptic ulcer, tension headache, asthma are good symptoms to take up for practising probing questions.

CHAPTER

3

Listening Skills

"We hear half of what is said, listen to half of what we hear, understand half of it, believe half of it and remember half of that."

—Anonymous

INTRODUCTION

Patients want to feel that the physician is working *with* them and *for* them, a kind of partner in health care who keeps patients' interest in the forefront. Several studies have shown that effective doctor-patient communication is the key to making them feel this way. It is also clear that *effective listening is often the missing link* in a dyad. We do ask many questions to the patients but quite often, we do not bother to listen fully to what they try to say.

Poor listening can hurt and hurt quite badly. Hundreds of errors in diagnosis and treatment can be traced down to poor listening. Once, a physician ordered Isoptin (verapamil) and the nurse concerned administered Isopril (isoprenaline) with disastrous result. Another example: A teenage girl who self-inflicted pin pricks to bleed from the ear (pinna) and nose was referred to many specialists and underwent several tests. All the wasteful expense could have been avoided if one had spent time listening to the details of bizarre bleeding episodes and the fact that this was the only way she could get the attention and sympathy from her tough father. Any health care professional will have dozens of similar anecdotes to narrate.

Any one who is not deaf can hear but listening is a skill that requires training, commitment and concentration. Table 3.1 summarises the differences between both.

In short, listening is hearing with a purpose; it is selective, focussed and an active process.

THE BENEFITS OF LISTENING

Rapport Building

Rapport is a close relationship usually one of mutual trust and emotional harmony. Listening to a patient helps develop rapport. Given a choice, patients will always consult a physician with

Table 3.1: Differences in hearing and listening

Hearing	*Listening*
Pure physical function	Mental and emotional experience involving logic and feelings
Simple activity of the central nervous system	Complex activity requiring translation, analysis, interpretation and evaluation
Effortless and automatic	Requires attention and concentration
Biological function of nature	Learned and cultivated skill
Can take in the sounds and noises simultaneously	Isolates sounds looking for meaning
Easy and can be relaxing	Can be difficult and tiring
Every one who can, hears	Only a few are good listeners
Is a prerequisite for listening but has no intrinsic value to it	Usually done with a motive like gathering information, enjoyment

whom they have rapport. Rapport building is therefore an important element of doctor-patient relationship.

Good rapport can make the patient-

- More willing to give you confidential information
- More likely to get things done by you
- More apt to get involved in your plan of management
- Less likely to reject treatment advice.

Information Gathering

The goal of a doctor-patient dyad is to glean a tremendous amount of *relevant* information. If patients perceive that the doctor is not listening, they may clam up, remain cool and reticent, rush through the consultation, or may mislead by giving incorrect historical details. On the other hand, strong listening by us makes them co-operative, volunteer important details, enjoy the dyad and take an active role in planning management.

Image Building

Patients label a physician, who is a good listener, as being *caring, considerate, kind, trustworthy, tactful, sincere, open minded, perceptive, intelligent, rational, ethical, humble, friendly, relaxed, forgiving* and *conscientious.*

On the contrary, a physician, who is a poor listener, may be labelled as being *aggressive, opinionated, hasty, arrogant, aloof, moody, uncaring, brash* or *absent-minded.*

These results from many studies should be enough to motivate all of us to be better listeners and enhance our image. It is very important in the early stages of one's career.

Persuading the Patient

A patient convinced against his/her will remains unconvinced. Studies have shown that one of the best ways to persuade others is by listening to their points first. Effective counsellors know this. They go on listening to a client's point of view until the client is ready to make his/her own decision.

Defusing Tension

Studies have shown that in tense situations, when clients are angry or upset, listening without arguing reduces tension in a few minutes. Arguing with an angry patient only aggravates the anger and is counterproductive.

OBSTACLES TO LISTENING

Since listening requires effort, concentration and attention, several obstacles may hinder listening. Some of the important obstacles are listed below. If one is aware of them, one could find ways of circumventing them.

Physical Setting

Noise, clutter, other people moving in and out, poor lighting, heat, humidity, overcrowded consulting room, etc. can all be major obstacles to listening. Better planning of the consulting rooms and of hospital working arrangements are ways of circumventing such obstacles.

Feelings About the Patient

These tend to affect our attention and keenness to listen to him/her. We see every person and thing through our own set of values. Differences in age, sex, race, education, cultural and social background, language, personal habits and beliefs can create difficulties in effective listening. Of course, these cut both ways. A patient who perceives great differences in his/her background will also have difficulties in listening to the physician.

The ways of circumventing such obstacles are, to develop an open mind, learn to accept variety as the spice of life, and to cultivate *professionalism*, i.e. effective performance at all times despite difficulties.

Bias Towards the Topic or Problem

If a patient and a physician hold opposite views, it may be impossible to converse. A common example is a patient who insists on his astrologer fixing the date and time for his surgery while his surgeon has no faith in astrology and is unwilling to let others dictate his surgical schedule. At times, the negative bias towards a problem may arise out of years of dealing with such problem cases. A common example is *irritable bowel syndrome*, which is very challenging and tiresome to manage. Many physicians develop a strong negative bias to this syndrome. They may have difficulty in listening to a new patient with 'the same old boring problem.'

The ways of circumventing such obstacles are, to develop patient centred outlook in medical practice, to develop tolerance to patients' idiosyncrasies, and to try to find out the secret of self-renewal.

Negative Messages from Patients

Some patients complain to the physician or criticise the health care facilities endlessly. This may put off the physician. Such behaviour is generally due to past experiences of patients.

Once this is realised, physician can empathise with such behaviour and reassure the patient appropriately during the current dyad. Handled thus, many 'grumpy patients' may turn a new leaf and become ardent fans of the 'great doctor'.

Indifference or Boredom

In India, this is a major reason as hospitals are terribly over crowded and patients throng the hospitals forming endless queues. Seeing the thirtieth case of 'irritable bowel' or 'tension headache' is enough to dump an unprepared physician into an abyss of boredom or indifference. Taking a quick break or mixing up different types of cases may help maintain interest.

Condition of the Listener

Physical, mental and emotional condition of the listener may be compromised due to over work, lack of sleep, minor illness or pre-occupation with more serious cases. To circumvent this, a physician has to first learn to "Listen to oneself." Doctors are notoriously poor in this but with practice, it is possible to recognise one's own limitation and circumvent them.

Physician Behaviour

Physicians are no angels. They too have their idiosyncratic behaviours that obstruct listening. Some of the common shortcomings are described below.

- *Mind Reading* is a common failure, especially among senior physicians. They tend to read too much into the patient's mind.
- *Labelling* a patient prematurely as "another case of xyz" short-circuits the interview process and leads to missed or wrong diagnosis. This happens with common symptoms reported by patients with less common diseases; aches and pains or lethargy in hypothyroidism, and headache or backache in giant cell arteritis are good examples. One may see a hundred cases of non-specific myalgia for every case of hypothyroidism but that is no excuse to label every hypothyroid as non-specific myalgia.
- *Premature counselling* is common. An asthmatic patient who said he worked in a cotton mill was counselled on the hazards of cotton dust. Out of politeness, he listened attentively until the end before saying that he worked in the computer room of the mill, which was dust free.
- *Rehearsing* the next question to ask even as the patient is answering the previous one is a sure way of not listening.
- *Scoring points* over the patient is the way of many insecure or diffident physicians. One should realise that a professional is expected to know more about a disease than a client does; therefore, showing off one's knowledge does not 'score any point'. Playing one-upmanship game is unprofessional and unethical and may also lead to errors of judgement.
- *Verbal duelling* is yet another method of putting down patients by engaging them in an argument.
- *Side stepping* the patient's concerns by using clichés like, "do not bother about it" or "grin and bear it" may put off the patient and abort the listening process.

EFFECTIVE LISTENING

If we were supposed to talk more than we listen, we would have two mouths and one ear.
—Mark Twain

It is worth repeating that we take listening for granted. Ineffective listening stems from poor listening habits or an assumption that "I do not have any problems in listening". Effective listening is a complex activity comprising of many elements and nearly everyone has weakness of one or more of the elements. Another reason is the common misperception that the responsibility for effective communication is with the speaker and not the listener. This is like holding the mouthpiece of a telephone responsible when the receiver goes *dead*.

Components of Listening

Four elements constitute the process of listening:

i. Physical hearing
ii. Understanding the meaning
iii. Analysing, verifying and weighing the information
iv. Determining an appropriate response.

One has to initially practise and strengthen each component and then put them together until effective listening becomes a habit.

Tips for Effective Listening

The following techniques, if mastered, can make you an effective listener:

1. Make a commitment to pay attention and listen.
   - Work to improve listening during medical and social interactions.
   - Prepare yourself, a) *mentally* by concentrating on listening, b) *physically* by proximity, reducing distractions like noise, etc. and c) *emotionally* by judging the worth of the information, not the speaker.
   - Realise that every speaker is entitled to his/her own opinion.
2. Do not interrupt; do not finish someone's sentence unless help is sought.
3. Avoid changing the topic midway by interrupting. At times, both play this game resulting in two *parallel monologues* or *pseudo dyad*. This results in zero listening.
4. Do not fake listening. It is rude. If you day dream or lose attention, it is better to ask the speaker to repeat.
5. Do not handle two or three other activities while listening. You can hear but not really listen if other activities distract you.
6. Use reflective phrases ('I see', etc.) and sentiments; use encouraging body language like nodding, eye contact, etc.
7. Develop the following *etiquette of listening*:
   - Give a 2 to 4-second pause between listening and responding, much longer than the normal response latency of 0.5 sec. This longish *inter response boundary* slows the pace of dyad and relaxes both.
   - Suppress the urge to *correct* wrong or misguided opinions.
   - Suppress the urge to rush and fill in silent pauses. Experience has shown that it is during pauses that many patients come out with vital information regarding their illness.
   - Close the present topic of discussion before changing to a new topic.

8. Use *empathic listening*. Feel *with* the patients. Avoid casual remarks on sensitive topics. Show support and reassurance by words or gestures. (*See below*)
9. Go for the main ideas and over all meaning. Analyse and evaluate: "What is she saying? Why is she saying it? How is she saying it? What does it all convey?" The pace of human speech is about 100 words per minute (wpm) but our intellect can process 600 to 1000 wpm. You should utilise this extra time to analyse what is being said by words, tone and gestures. This is called *active listening*.
10. Listen for vague and incomplete information and for important clues. Speaker *knows* what he is trying to say but the listener may not comprehend its implication easily.

    Once, a stoic patient with *non-specific myalgia* consulting the fifth hospital in 2 years was about to be sent off with reassurance when he casually remarked, "I can eat *Idli* but not *Chappatti*." The smart young resident was intrigued and resumed his interview. The difficulty in chewing tough food turned out to be due to myasthenia. But for this cue recognition, the diagnosis would have certainly been delayed by a few more months. Experienced physicians can perhaps remember several such *vital clues* casually dropped by their patients that turned out to be of great importance in the diagnosis and management of cases.
11. Verify what the qualifying adjectives used by patients mean: "how big is *big*?" "how frequent is *often*" "how much is *expensive* for you?"
12. Listen and look for *acceptance signals* (openness, visible smile, coming closer, etc.) that indicate that the patient is likely to adhere to your advice and follow the plan of management.

ADVANCED SKILLS: EMPATHIC LISTENING

Listening and empathising are essential skills when relating to others. Empathy means understanding another person so well that you identify with him/her, you feel like he/she does. It is listening so intently and identifying so closely that you experience the other person's situation, thoughts and emotions. Good clinicians do this, so do good friends.

Purposes

- It shows that you care and that you understood the patient. S/he will prefer talking to you and will be more open.
- If you misunderstand the patient, s/he can immediately correct your impressions.
- It directs the conversation towards important emotional issues close to the patient.
- It lets the patient know that you (the listener) accept him/her and are ready to listen to personal details. It invites him/her to tell his/her story and vent his/her feelings.
- Since it is safe to talk about "deep" subjects like fears and phobias or hopes and aspirations, a patient can express feelings and self-explore, considering all his/her deep-seated emotions and motives. Thus, it is therapeutic.
- It reduces our irritation with patients' behaviour because we understand. *To understand is to accept and to forgive.*
- It may reduce our prejudice about our patients and improve our tolerance because we realise what kind of persons they really are. Furthermore, we discover that everyone is "understandable."
- It fosters a more meaningful, closer and fiduciary relationship with our patients.

Cultivating Empathy Skills

Empathy is one of the more important skills one will ever acquire. It is amazing how few professionals do it well.

i. Learn to be a good, active listener (See above).
ii. Understand what is involved in empathy responding.

Empathy is conveyed by letting the patient know that we have understood. It is even more complex than listening. You do not have to be perfect, but the more accurate an empathiser you are, the better. A good empathiser focuses on the speaker's feelings and not on his/her actions or circumstances. *Example*: When talking with someone whose parent has died, do not ask, "What happened?" or "When?" but instead attend to and reflect the feelings, "It really hurts" or "Do you feel abandoned and lost." When one is upset, one needs to handle one's feelings before one can concentrate on solving the problems and empathy helps in achieving this.

Levels of Empathy Response

First Level: Inaccurate Reflection or Distracting Comments

Most doctor-patient dyads are examples of this level. The common ploys used by us to avoid empathising are described below using the example of a hypertensive patient who feels "uneasy" after starting on treatment.

- *Changing-the-topic responses*: When the patient complains about a troublesome side effect of therapy, you just say, "Your BP is better now."
- *"I know better than you" response*: These are god-like pronouncements, such as "There's nothing wrong with the treatment. You will feel better tomorrow."
- *Judgmental responses*: Passing value judgement like, "Good patients tolerate minor side effects; they do not run to the doctor like a cry baby."
- *Advising* response: Parental advice on what could be done, e.g. "If the medicine causes problems, do not take it. We shall change over to some other medicine." This solves the problem but without conveying any empathy.
- *Discounting* and *premature reassurance*: "Oh, everybody has side effects, do not worry about it. You will get over it." This is saying, "Do not talk to me about it any more." (Also called 'smooth talk').
- *Psychoanalysing*: "You are a nervous person worried about adverse reactions all the time."
- *By-passing questions*: "Do you have nausea? Do you have vomiting? Did you have diarrhoea? No? Then do not say side effect." (These circumvent the patient's concern about "feeling uneasy." Such questions are used in clinical dyads to control patients from talking more about it.)
- *Blowing your own trumpet*: "See, when I took the same treatment I got..." (this is not so bad, if you remember to return to your patient's concern.)

Most of us are guilty of some of these unempathic responses. A few poor responses occasionally are no problem, but many of us are 'instant reassurers' and 'constant questioners'. We tend to dispose of our patient's problems in 3-5 minutes. A significant problem may take several minutes to hours spent over a few dyads to be of any help.

Second Level: Partly Understanding of the Patient's Feelings

At this level, the listener does not entirely understand the patient's feelings. This may discourage the patient from expressing more feelings unless the listener indicates an interest. Suppose a patient tells you how badly he misses his cigarettes and you respond, "Yes, it often happens. So do you want to go back to bad habits?" He may reply, "Oh, no, I am not that stupid!" You have empathised a little with withdrawal pangs but you have not elicited his true feelings. It is usually our emotional reactions to what has been said that causes our misunderstandings (see "crossed transaction").

Third Level: An Accurate Empathy Response that Captures the Patient's Feelings

You have put yourself "in their shoes." Your comments reflect exactly what the patient has told you. Then the patient knows you are attending closely and that you care. But be brief. Use simple words and use your own words (paraphrasing); otherwise, you may sound like a "parrot" to him/her. It is important to make frequent comments reflecting your understanding of what has just been said. If the patient gets no comment from you for two or three minutes, s/he may conclude that you do not understand, approve or care. When you show accurate empathy, the patient appears visibly aroused and usually says, "Exactly, doctor" or words to that effect.

Fourth Level: Adding to the Patient's Self-understanding

It is possible for an astute listener to understand (guess) what a patient is feeling even before s/he has recognised or expressed his/her own emotion. For example, to a patient who appears anxious, as soon as you suggest to him/her if s/he might be feeling anxious about something, s/he may readily recognise the underlying emotion, accept your interpretation and say, "Exactly, doctor." This can add greatly to the patient's insight, awareness or understanding of his/her feelings and the situation.

Caution: Interpretations are always guesses, so be tentative and ask indirect, non-leading questions like, "Could it be..." or "I'm wondering if...", etc.

Fifth Level: Fantastic Insight

After studying a patient well over a long time, one may be able to provide some brilliant insight occasionally. Great insight is a rare event. Even highly experienced clinicians offer profound, creative insights only on occasions. It requires both an open-minded patient and a creative empathic doctor. The non-verbal behaviour of the patient faithfully reveals the emotional component of the patient's message. Once we learn how to tune into it, we can develop insight into the true feelings of the patient (see Neuro-linguistic programming).

iii. Practice giving empathic responses

With experience, you will learn to be better at guessing about the patient's feelings. These derive from three major sources:

Listen to the Patient

a. Hear the spoken words and tone of voice, but, also, observe his/her facial expression and other non-verbal messages. Read "between the lines" for subtle suggestions of feelings.

b. Remember any hints about possible causes of his/her feelings, e.g. a comment that his/her friend died recently may indicate the source of anxiety.

Listen to Your Own Reactions

a. Place yourself mentally in the patient's situation; then imagine what you would do and how you would feel. This is one of the most powerful techniques for generating "intuition" about the patient's emotions.
b. If you have had experiences similar to that of the patient, then you can recall and mentally recreate the feelings you had. It is reasonable to assume that the talker may also feel the same way.

Make Use of Your Memory

You have a general notion about how other patients with problems similar to that of the present patient have responded. This accumulated wisdom grows as you create a mental bank of case studies, and have more life experience. The mental bank may help in empathising with the patient.

Problems in Empathic Listening

Although empathising is an excellent way to respond when someone has a problem, there are pitfalls when using the method and misconceptions about the method:

- When you empathise, you are inviting the patient to become emotional. Do not do that unless you are *genuinely* interested in helping the patient.
- There is a possibility that the patient will feel worse after talking about and reviewing his/her problems. This is especially true of depressed and angry patients.
- Sometimes empathy works so well that a doctor starts to use empathic response excessively, turning even casual conversation into a deep therapeutic session. Skills as a light conversationalist are also needed.
- The patient may erroneously assume that your accurate reflection of his/her feelings means that you agree with his/her opinions or morals. Occasionally (not always), you may feel the need to correct his/her misunderstanding. This should be done briefly. *Example*: If a truck driver tells you about his high-risk behaviour and his concern about getting HIV-AIDS, you might say, "Yes, yes. Any one would feel concerned about that and I understand how you feel." Nevertheless, he should not go away feeling that you approve of his high-risk behaviour.
- Many beginners think it easy to empathise—all one has to do is *sympathise*. This is not true. You have to detect the unspoken feelings, communicate your understanding, and provide new insights. In addition, there may be behaviours, e.g. paedophilia, which may be so wrong, so immoral, or so disgusting to you that you may not be able to empathise.
- The accuracy of your empathy response can not be judged until your patient responds, indicating if he/she thinks you have understood. If s/he does not agree with your observation or interpretation, you get a low empathy rating.

Empathy responding is one of the better-researched treatment methods. It has been demonstrated to be and effective way for doctors to respond in a therapeutic relationship. There are a cluster of traits associated with being empathic, such as having unconditional positive regard, being genuine, warm, open, specific and concrete, self-disclosing and so on. It is an art that is honed over a lifetime of clinical practice.

SUMMARY

To sum up, if questioning and answering form the 'efferent' limb of communication, listening is the 'afferent' limb. Both the limbs need to be strengthened for effective communication to take place.

BIBLIOGRAPHY

1. Active listening available at http://www.mindtools.com/CommSkll/ActiveListening.htm.
2. Internet has excellent resources on empathy training http://www.mindtools.com/CommSkll/EmphaticListening.htm; http://wilderdom.com/games/PsychologicalExercises.html.
3. Nichols MP. *The lost art of listening*. San Luis Obispo, CA: Impact Publishers, 1995.
4. Slesinski RA. Effective listening. *How to skyrocket your sales*. UBSPD, New Delhi, 1995.

PRACTICAL EXERCISES

Microtraining of Component Skills in Effective Listening

To learn complex skills like listening, one needs to use component skill training, also known as 'microtraining.' Students listen to simulated patients and practise one component at a time viz.,

i. Removing obstacles to listening
ii. Active listening
iii. Etiquette of listening
iv. Conveying empathy
v. Clarifying vague information (reading 'between lines' and 'beyond lines').

During the simulated dyad, each student's performance is observed with the help of a checklist, by his/her peers and by the tutor. A detailed feedback session follows in which the individual performances are constructively criticised. Repeated practice can be arranged until all the students attain minimum expected competence.

Role-play Simulation

Once the students acquire basic component skills, full-scale simulation role-play can be arranged in which dyads between the students and simulated patients takes place. Peers and tutors observe using a rating scale to assess the performance of each student. Formative feedback is given in the end. If feasible, video recording followed by feedback session will be a more effective training method.

Listening for Feelings

First, talk about listening for feelings. Make a list of feelings. Start with *mad, sad, bad, glad*. Ask them to work in small groups and write down 10 to 20 situations that will make them feel that way.

Play audiotapes and videotapes of short segments of conversations from films and TV serials that convey different shades of emotions and feelings. Use gross skits first, which are easily sorted as one of the four emotional labels. Then move on to mixed emotions when students realise that sad, mad, bad and glad are not enough to classify finer shades of feelings.

There are plenty of doctor-patient dyads in films. One can easily compile about 20 segments from them and conduct this session.

Empathy Training

Role-play: Students form into groups of three. Each one takes turns being:

1. The listener giving empathic responses,
2. The talker pretending to have a variety of problems and
3. The assessor giving feedback to the empathiser using the 14-item empathy checklist using a 3-point scale
   (0 = not done; 1= partially done; 2 = well done).

Empathy Checklist

1. Display true concern and interest in the patient's situation.
2. Use affirming and reassuring statements to connect with patients.
3. Maintain a high-level of active listening throughout the conversation, even during emotional outbursts.
4. Use "I" or "We" statements.
5. Use "Yes" statements frequently ("Sure, let's take a look at that.")
6. Avoid "No" statements.
7. Pick up on trigger statements that signal problems and issues.
8. Whenever appropriate, probe to uncover the root cause behind the patient's questions.
9. Convey reasons behind your probing questions.
10. Whenever appropriate, paraphrase the patient's statement and check for accurate understanding.
11. Use appropriate emotional responses that reflect the patient's situation.
12. Acknowledge the patient's feelings by reflective statements ("It sounds like you are upset about this.")
13. Express positive reactions when patient is pleased with your service.
14. Carry out all actions committed to the patient.

Debriefing is done in a plenary session where experiences of all the groups are shared. Any doubts are clarified by the tutor.

Micro-training for skills involved in empathic behaviour: Using 'microteaching' techniques, micro-training for *Skills Involved in Empathic Behaviour* can be conducted. Each student gets to practise a pre-determined component skill in empathic behaviour for 5 to 10 minutes. The observers and simulated patients give a component specific feedback using the following rating scale:

Rating Scale to Assess Empathy*

Eye Contact

1. Little or no eye contact
2. Some eye contact

**Reference:* Deladisma AM, Cohen M, Stevens A, et al. Do medical students respond empathetically to a virtual patient? The Amer J Surg. 2007;193:756–60.

3. Appropriate eye contact at most times
4. Appropriate eye contact at all times

Head Nod

1. Little or no head nodding
2. Some head nodding
3. Appropriate head nodding at most times
4. Appropriate head nodding at all times

Body Lean

1. Little or no forward body lean
2. Some forward body lean
3. Appropriate forward lean at most times
4. Appropriate forward lean at all times

Immersion Level

1. Did not appear to be immersed at anytime
2. Appeared to be immersed some of the time
3. Appeared to be immersed most of the time
4. Appeared to be immersed at all times

Anxiety

1. Appeared anxious at all times
2. Appeared anxious at most times
3. Had some anxiety during the interview
4. Little or no anxiety

Attitude

1. Made judgmental comments, criticized patient; *OR* talked down to patient
2. Made 1-2 comments within appropriate affect
3. No judgmental comments; talk to patient as an equal
4. No judgmental comments; talked to patient as equal and offered praise/encouragement when opportunity arose

Question Clarity

1. Frequent unclear questions; patient had difficulty in understanding what was being asked
2. Some unclear questions; patient had difficulty once or twice understanding what was being asked
3. Mostly clear questions
4. Clear questions

Empathy Rating

1. Offered no empathetic comments; No encouragement or support (did not state intention to help)
2. Offered only brief supportive or empathetic comments and only in response to a distinct emotional statement by patient; comments may seem prospective or forced.
3. Offered empathetic or supportive comments *OR* stated intention to help
4. Offered empathetic or supportive comments *OR* stated intention to help; despite limited time, seemed to be on the way to establishing a caring relationship

Overall Rating

1. Very unsatisfactory
2. Unsatisfactory
3. Satisfactory
4. Superior
5. Outstanding

CHAPTER

4

Non-verbal Behavior (NVB)

What we are communicates far more eloquently than anything we Say or Do.
—S Covey

INTRODUCTION

Whenever two persons talk to each other directly, the meaning of a message is not merely derived from the spoken words but from an amalgamation of the following:

- Spoken word - Language
- Voice tone - Para-language
- Gesture and expression- Body-language
- Dress and grooming - Personal appearance, e.g. over-coat, hairstyle, etc.
- Possessions - Personal effects, e.g. pen, stethoscope, etc.
- Affiliation and activity - Context and intent of the behavior.

Ray Birdwhistell, an anthropologist, has estimated that during a typical dyad, only one-third of the message is conveyed by spoken words; the rest is conveyed by the other elements of communication. Albert Mehrabian, in 'Silent Messages,' has said that spoken words carried only 7% of feelings, emotions and attitudes, para-language, 38%, and body language, the remaining 55%. Truly then, *action speaks louder than words.*

DEFINITION

Body language includes any voluntary, involuntary or reflex movement of a part, or all of the body. This communicates emotional messages to the outside world. These signals are often missed or misread unless a person is trained in socio-cultural nuances of body language. In contrast, non-verbal behavior (NVB) includes body language and all the other non-verbal cues like appearance, possessions and affiliations.

LISTENING WITH THE EYES

The total message conveyed during any dyad includes facts, ideas, principles, feelings, attitudes, values, self-concept, needs, aspirations and motivation. A listener may not receive many of these if s/he is *blind* to the non-verbal signals and *deaf* to the verbal ones.

Non-verbal signals are subconscious, unless the person is an actor playing a role. Usually these gestures just precede the verbal output and one has to train oneself to look for these signs at that point of time. After taking ward rounds for years with students and residents, I am convinced that the most important difference between a senior clinician and a novice is the ability to perceive and interpret NVB.

There are about 5000 gestures using the hands and 20,000 using the face. One should look for the *big picture* and understand the main message than analyse gestures in isolation.

When verbal and non-verbal messages are contradictory, one instinctively tends to believe the latter. Research has proven this valid. It is easy for the conscious mind to utter falsehood by words. On the contrary, it is virtually impossible for the subconscious mind, which controls spontaneous gestures and expressions, to lie. Moreover, the involuntary non-verbal output always precedes the conscious verbal output. Physicians, who appear to have great insight into patients' minds, are generally adept at picking up these true non-verbal messages from them.

Clinicians assessing mental status interpret patients' non-verbal behavior in terms of its i) quantum of discharge, ii) expression, iii) interactional cues, and iv) neurological signs like Parkinsonism, Bell's palsy, etc. While decoding non-verbal expression for interactional cues, consider the three general aspects discussed below. These contribute to forming an initial impression. One should also look for the major NVB signals described later.

READING AND RESPONDING TO MAJOR NON-VERBAL SIGNALS

Individual signs of body language, though important, may not convey the whole picture and at times, may even mislead. The 'big picture' has to be taken into account. The cumulative meaning of NVB may be classified into the following eight non-verbal signals. Once understood, it is easier for a physician to follow the signals emitted by a patient and respond appropriately.

Closed versus Open Position

Fear, nervousness, scepticism, defensiveness, secretiveness, confusion, lack of rapport and similar negative emotions result in closed signs. Some of the universal signs of *closed position* are:

- A hand over the mouth
- The arms folded tightly across the chest
- Hugging an object (a book or a hand-bag) or clutching it with both hands
- Locked legs or interlocked big toes
- Lack of eye contact, tense or blank expression, and covering the face.

In *sari*-clad women, *"pallu sign"* (*pallu* is the extra length of sari, normally covering the chest and hanging free at the back is wrapped around to cover the whole upper torso) is a strong sign of closed position. In some communities, *pallu* is used to cover the head also. A common variation of this sign is tugging the right border of sari in front of the chest in an attempt to cover the front torso better. Less common are tugging the left border and tucking it in to the waist line. Similar signs can also be perceived with other dresses like skirt and *salwar-kameez* (tugging at the hem of a skirt and readjusting the *duppatta*).

Outstretched arms, open relaxed limbs, loose smooth motion, legs standing at ease (comfortably apart), friendly face and comfortable eye contact are the hallmarks of *open position*. Undoing signs of closed position, e.g. unlocking the big toes or re-adjusting the sari also indicate open position.

Caution

These 'open signs' indicate a confidant, fearless, clear-headed state and imply trust in the attending physician. Young male doctors should not misread these signals in female patients as having sexual undertone. Such errors can lead to wrong responses, which are unprofessional misdemeanours and unethical acts.

Possessions and Appearance

The way people dress and appear make statements on their lifestyle, beliefs and the state of health. Men from rural India shave only once in a few days and only if they feel well. Therefore, *the beard sign* often indicates ill health in them. One of my favourite quote is, "A beard—with fever and a heart lesion is infective endocarditis, with haemoptysis is pulmonary TB, with jaundice is viral hepatitis, with epigastric pain is active peptic ulcer and with pain in the right upper quadrant is amoebic liver abscess." New residents from other states are surprised until they realise that all these unrelated conditions are subacute problems and common in south India; these affect the sense of well being and then the rural men stop shaving.

Similarly, *mehndi* application on the fingertips or nail polish in rural women and men indicate festivities or celebrations. From the proximal length of new nail growth, one can even guess when the event took place. This is not a mere curiosity. Our studies on non-adherence to therapy have shown that among patients, who have chronic problems such as diabetes mellitus, hypertension or heart disease, festivities as well as grievances are major reasons for skipping therapy.

Some other *appearance signals* in India are new bangles, dress or footwear, and shaved head. The last sign, especially in females, indicates a religious pilgrimage and the hair growth can say when it took place. In males, it could also be due to death of a parent or a first degree relative. A newly married woman is often detected by her shiny new jewels, silver anklet with noisy bells and too ostentatious a dress for medical consultation. "Honeymoon cystitis" and early pregnancy are common reasons for such consultations.

Distance and Direction

Turning towards and moving closer to the other person are open positive signs except when aggressive in intent. Turning around and moving away are signs of withdrawal. Turning at right angles could be a *warm* or *cold* sign depending on if the person was initially facing away or not. Instead of the whole person moving, only the upper torso or the face may reveal these signs.

Language Proficiency and Hand Movement

Stammering and gesturing is often seen in our patients when they try to speak in English rather than their mother tongue. A study found that bilingual subjects speaking in their non-dominant language produced more groping hand movements and stammer more. In addition, in comparison with a high imagery (picturesque) topic, when the subjects spoke about a low imagery (non-picturesque) topic, they displayed more pointing movements. Clinicians listening to bilingual patients may wrongly interpret an increase in motor activity as a sign of psychopathology (Marcos, 1979).

Touching and Self-Concept

Persons with low self-concept, who are unsure of themselves, touch their body more frequently than those with a high self-concept (Muller et al, 1980). If doctors want to project an image of confidence, they should avoid touching themselves while talking to the patients (or their examiners!).

The following paragraphs describe eight major non-verbal signals and suggest how to respond to them if you perceive them in your patients.

Positive Signals

These indicate agreement, enthusiasm or co-operation. These are seen in those patients with whom you already have a good rapport or when the dyad is proceeding in a way that patients appreciate much.

- Nodding, smiling, alert and relaxed face
- *Sprinter's position* of sitting on the edge of the seat, leaning forwards with feet on tip toes and a slight tilt of the head (even pet dogs do this!)
- Fully attentive with riveting eye contact and without any hostility
- Rubbing the palms together
- Coat or vest unbuttoned, sleeves rolled up, *pallu* of *sari* gathered and tucked in to the waistline.
- Open body position
- Standing at ease—legs comfortably apart with hands on the hip

The following indicate inclination to further interaction:

- Changed voice-tone—gentler and conciliatory, or more animated and enthusiastic
- Body positioning—moving closer, tilting head towards, or aligning the shoulder towards you
- Hand gestures: rub, clap, pat, grab, touch or shake hands.

How to Respond

- Show appreciation by gestures or smiling; thank him/her when appropriate.
- Note the things you say or do (*"hot-buttons"*) that elicit positive signals from the patient; continue in the same vein to build an even better rapport. For example, if mention of non-drug therapy elicits such a response from your patient, spend more time explaining it further.
- Show friendliness and an equal enthusiasm; listen intently.
- Respond to any interactive gesture in an appropriate way with out crossing the ethical norms.

Thinking Signals

When a major decision has to be made by the patient and the options are many, a patient may show these signs:

- Repetitive gestures like rubbing the chin or neck, twisting the hair, scratching with a finger tip, tapping on the head, smoothening the hair, beard or moustache, etc.
- Chin resting on the palm while the thumb and fingers touch and stroke either cheek
- Meditating expression, look of concentration, intense but blank stare *at* the wall, ceiling or floor or *through* you
- Hands clasped *behind* the back with the head bent down and downcast eyes, or *thinker statue* like posture (flexed sitting position with forehead resting on the hand)
- Pinching the nose-bridge with eyes closed, rubbing the eyes or lips, or stroking the corners of the mouth; simpletons and small children may elaborately pick the nose or ear while in deep thought
- Methodically and slowly wiping spectacles, putting objects like a pencil or an ear-piece of spectacles in the mouth; a smoker may inhale deeply and others may take deep breaths
- Repeatedly mumbles to self or asks reassuring questions; doodles (scribbles) letters or an object repeatedly.

How to Respond

- Do not interrupt while the patient thinks deeply; keep looking at the face and wait for eye contact
- Elicit reasons for deep thinking: Is it due to wavering, being unsure or fear?
- Summarise major benefits of following your advice
- Anticipate and respond to any further queries
- Reassure on how good the decision would be; use facts and figures, not jokes or frivolous remarks.

Caution

Some of these signs may be due to boredom and a patient may let his/her thoughts wander to other concerns. Beware! Double check by eliciting some responses from the patient.

Signals of Disinterest and Restlessness

The following signals suggest boredom or disinterest. Patients show these when one tries to advise them an unacceptable treatment option like giving up smoking.

- Blank, *zombie* like expression that looks through you
- Avoidance of eye-contact or drooping eyelids
- Absent verbal or non-verbal response
- Repeated yawning
- Chin resting on hands, body slouched in seat with legs stretched out
- Body and head turned away
- In a group, talking among themselves, sharing jokes or passing notes around (diversion).

Caution

Remember that these signs may also indicate underlying fatigue or sleepiness. In that case, fix another appointment.

The following signs indicate **restlessness**. These are more often seen in a doctor than a patient! So check yourself if you inadvertently reveal these signs!.

- Fidgeting in the seat or couch
- Restless gestures like tapping, drumming, looking at the wristwatch repeatedly, clicking a ball pen, etc.
- Crossed legs with one foot kicking or tapping
- Frequent nodding and hastening the dyad
- Doodling, bending clips, or tearing slips of paper.

How to Respond

- Ask relevant questions and force attention and interaction
- Skim over 'boring' topics and focus on areas of interest to the patient; alternately stress why the apparently boring information is of importance to the patient
- Create interest using humour, drama, anecdotes or facts in an enthusiastic, involved and interactive way
- Take a break and resume later.

Confidence Signals

These are often seen in VIP cases and persons who have been in positions of authority. The *tough ones* (in my experience) are village headmen, elderly schoolteachers, head priests and heads of organisations. They may show the following signs:

- Stand or sit erect
- Lean back on the seat with hands on the back of the head
- Facial expression of inner calm and poise
- Lack of nervous mannerisms
- Frequent direct eye contact
- Joining the fingertips in front—the *steeple gesture*; higher the steeple gesture, more is the feeling of superiority; an extreme case may peer at you through the steeple hands!
- Speaking slowly, in a lower pitch and a relaxed manner.

How to Respond

- A good way to say that you are on the patient's side is to acknowledge his experience or expertise and that you are glad to be of service to him/her (see "superior personality")
- Do not get intimidated; the other person may be great in his/her own field but then you are a professional too and your help has been deemed necessary by the other person
- Act confident yourself but do not try to challenge; it is unprofessional and may also stir *the hornet's nest* and divert the attention from health care concerns
- Subtly reveal your knowledge, expertise and professionalism thereby establishing your credibility; after all you should know more than the patient on health care issues of your speciality.

Signals of Scepticism

A patient who has doubts, disbelief, confusion or distrust may reveal these signs. It is commonly seen when there is a mismatch between *illness* and *disease*. Illness is what the patient perceives and disease is what the doctor perceives. Many 'severe illnesses' may just be 'trivial diseases' and *vice-versa.* If the doctor is not empathetic in such situations, a patient is bound to show the following signs.

- Raised eyebrows and a quick sideways glance (I find it more in female patients)
- Facial expressions of frown, smirk, sarcasm or amazement
- Open mouth with finger on the lower teeth or finger tapping on the chin; shaking of the head sideways
- Scratching the head or rubbing the nose
- Pushing back in a chair, stepping back or turning away on a couch with defensive crossing of arms
- (Patients wearing glasses) Lowering the spectacles and peering over them at the ceiling or the floor.

How to Respond

- Empathise with the patient; elicit reasons for doubt and clarify with ample proof from authoritative sources
- Fully explain any illness-disease paradoxes to promote understanding
- Use open, friendly position and positive gestures
- If the patient seems unconvinced, *agree to disagree* until the next dyad.

Negative Signals

A patient with feelings of hostility, anger or frustration may show these signs:

- Increased eye contact with a challenging look, squinted glance, taut face and frowning expression
- Closed body-position with clenching of fists or clutching the edge of a table, chair or couch
- *The self-controlling gestures*: A palm on the back of the neck and locked ankles; arms across the chest with fingers tightly clutching the upper arms
- Restless signals (see above)
- Abrupt, jerky movements and aggressive body shifts, banging on a table or a cot
- *Aggressive gestures*: Destroying small objects like paper clips and rubber bands or crushing a paper violently.

How to Respond

- Use non-threatening body postures and calm voice
- Elicit reasons for restlessness or anger
- If anger is 'at something else', allow it to be let off. Studies have shown that giving time to vent anger and frustration helps soothe the person in a few minutes; the person may in fact smile at you at the end of it!
- Never inflame the patient by arguing or vehemently denying
- If the patient 'does not get it', blame it on your inability to get it across effectively.

Caution

With a psychiatric case, or a very hostile person, keep a good distance, maintain eye-contact at all times, keep the door and windows open; call for help if things seem to go out of hand.

Signals of Deception

Patients do not always say what they think or feel; they often say what they think you wish to hear from them. The following signals should caution one not to take the patient's words at face value.

- *The Hot-seat syndrome*: Squirming in the seat, especially if the patient feels nervous about lying to the doctor or suspects that lying has been detected.
- *Nervous mannerisms*: Picking nails, finger tapping, playing with jewellery or pen, repeatedly readjusting the specs on the nose, or *the pallu of a sari* or *duppatta*; frequent smacking or licking of the lips; repeatedly wiping the face with hand or a kerchief; wringing of hands, especially when pressed to answer
- *Voice changes*: High pitched rapid speech at high volume; short and rapid breathing; unnecessary repetition or stammering
- *Self-comforting gestures*: Palm on the head, handclasp, etc.
- Eye contact goes to either extremes of a) avoiding direct eye-contact, throwing furtive sideways glance or looking up and down, and b) over compensated prolonged eye-contact with nodding of the head and tapping on the furniture, (*the believe me* gesture).
- Sudden non-purposive movements, especially when telling a lie
- *The double cross sign:* Cross arms defensively, then uncross while lying, and then cross again in a defensive or defiant way.

How to Respond

- Never imply that you know that the patient is lying and never directly challenge veracity, except in rare instances of a chronic defaulter, etc.
- Elicit response in different ways to check for veracity; it is difficult to lie consistently
- Correct their mistakes authoritatively with facts, figures and evidences; speak in a non-judgemental manner
- If you can not make the patient tell the truth, agree to disagree until the next dyad.

Signals of Hurry

These are more commonly seen among doctors than patients. If a patient is in a hurry to catch a bus or empty the bladder or bowel, or if s/he wants an unpleasant dyad to end, the following signals may be present:

- Signs of restlessness (see above *)
- Looking at the time frequently
- Answering even before the question is fully asked
- Short and curt responses even to open-ended queries
- Repeated attempts to get up from the chair
- If the meeting is accidental while crossing paths, not stopping but continuing to continue to walk, drive, etc.

How to Respond

- Confirm if the patient is in a hurry to attend to some thing else
- Fix up another convenient time to meet; if the message is urgent, ask for a minute and tell the gist.

SPECIFIC NON-VERBAL SIGNS IN PRACTICE

Many NVB signs have been described and are formally taught in the schools of drama and dance. These form the *words* and *phrases of the non-verbal language.* More relevant to us are the NVB signs studied in health care settings by various researchers. Some of the major findings are summarised in this section. These form the vocabulary of the body language.

The Eyes and The Face

Eye Contact

A physician should consider a variety of factors in evaluating the patient's eye contact including cultural background, emotional state, personality characteristics, and gender.

In a Japanese study (Bond and Komai, 1976), when the interviewer gazed at subjects' eyes, their response latencies were shortened and body movements were reduced, reflecting greater subject involvement in the interaction. When the subjects gazed at the interviewer's eyes, the subjects increased self-manipulation using their hands, reflecting the upsetting effects of monitoring the interviewer's face during interaction. The consequences of *gazing at another's eyes* thus appear to be different from *having one's eyes gazed at* by another.

If your patient seems to go rigid or answers questions with nervous rapidity, it indicates the intensity of patient's involvement in the dyad. You may gaze at the person less and even move away a little bit to give her more space. If the patient shows excessive self-manipulation while making eye contact with you, you may reduce the duration of eye contact to reduce upsetting her.

White of the Eye and Emotion

Exposed eye area (EEA) was measured in Indian adults who modelled six emotions, viz., happiness, sadness, fear, anger, surprise, disgust and a neutral expression. EEA for fear and surprise were significantly larger, and the EEA for disgust was significantly smaller than that for other emotions (Mandal, 1992). Beware of the narrowed palpabral fissure—it may indicate disgust.

Gazing and Personality

The duration of eye contact gives us an indication of the extraverted nature of the patient. A study of 20 extraverted and 20 introverted women found that the *extraverted women made longer eye contact while listening.* Gazing at the interviewer while speaking was similar in both groups. The women gazed longer at a female interviewer than at a male interviewer (Iizuka, 1992).

Facial Expression and Rapport-Building

Nonverbal interactions may contribute to development of a "visual holding environment" in its broadest sense. This may be based on mutual needs of the patient and the clinician to *hold and to be held.* It may be as difficult for a clinician as a patient to feel warm towards the other person who is blind to the non-verbal facial signals. The development of therapeutic relationship involves active and mutual eye contact, the *language of silence*. Facial expressions form a bridge to personal relatedness between the therapist and the patient (Weil, 1984-5).

The clinician's face therefore, has a crucial role in the development of therapeutic relationship. A patient can read and respond to the facial expressions of the clinician and build a therapeutically symbiotic relationship. During this phase, *either player's facial expressions "belong" as much to the other as to oneself* (Searles, 1984-5).

This study explains how some physicians can put off their patients forever by their unfriendly facial expressions and blindness to non-verbal signals of the patients.

Facial Expression of Type A Personality

In a study, facial expressions of 24 type A and 24 type B men were examined. Two expressions viz., *glare* and *disgust* significantly differentiated type A from type B. The Glare and Disgust scores in turn correlated most notably with hostility, which is associated with coronary artery disease (Chesney, 1990).

Omega Sign of Depression

The corrugator muscle region of the forehead has special significance in producing facial expressions associated with depression. Darwin observed in 1872 that contractions in the corrugator region produce peculiarly formed wrinkles on the forehead, referred to as *"Omega Melancholium."* In a study, 61 women with major depressive disorder showed a significant positive correlation between facial corrugator electromyographic values and psychomotor agitation. These data indicate that excessive corrugator muscle activity causes the *Omega sign* of melancholia and depression (Greden, 1985).

Facial Expression in Pain

Facial expressions contribute substantially to the judgement of sufferer's pain. In a study, volunteers' facial reactions to pain were analysed. The common facial actions were:

- Narrowing of the palpebral fissure from below,
- Raising the upper lip, pulling the lip corners, parting of the lips, or dropping the jaw, and
- Eyes closing or frequently blinking.

These reactions were most salient at the onset, expressing blends of startle, adaptive reaction and emotional reaction to pain. The relation between subjective distress and facial expression was greatest at the beginning of noxious stimulation; they declined in vigour over time, although self-report of pain continued to mount. The social models had a potent impact on verbal report and pain tolerance but not on facial expression, indicating relative independence of component reactions of painful experience (Craig, 1985).

This study corroborates with our every day hospital experience. When we judge pain merely by their facial expression, our patients 'seem to get used to the pain after some time'. This is not true; the pain continues to mount but as time passes by, their faces do not reflect it as well. We have to elicit verbal description to know how they feel. The exceptions are illiterate women of low economic status, whose social model permits them to continue to cry loudly, often using colourful phrases to describe their pain. This is most prominently seen and heard in our labour rooms.

Faking and Suppressing Pain

In a study of patients with chronic low back pain, the facial display of pain reflected differences between *sources* of pain, *social context* in which pain is induced and *individual differences* among patients. Considerable voluntary control over the facial expression of pain was observed (Prkachin, 1992). However, attempts to suppress the facial grimace of pain were not entirely successful.

The faked expression was more an intensified caricature of the genuine expression (Craig, 1991). In another study, assessors attributed more pain to those who faked pain than to those who suppressed their facial expression of pain (Poole, 1992). It is indeed difficult to guess if a grimace is faked caricature of pain or a true indicator of severe pain. It is safer to give the benefit of doubt to the patients until one learns more about their background.

Lie Detection

In a study, truth and falsehood were classified thus: sincere agreement or sincere disagreement (*truthful*), pretending to agree (*ingratiating lie*), and pretending to disagree (*non-ingratiating lie*). Observers then rated the sincerity of each message based on information available from one of four different channels: *verbal* (written words only), *audio* (audiotape only), *visual* (videotape without sound), and *audio-visual* (videotape with sound). Results showed that—

a. Lies told by women were more readily detected than lies told by men.
b. Lies told to the opposite sex were more easily detected than lies to same sex targets.
c. Ingratiating lies were more successfully detected than were non-ingratiating lies, particularly when told to attractive targets.
d. For ingratiating lies, detectability was greatest with videotapes (visual non-verbal cues).
e. Persons addressing an attractive listener were perceived as being less sincere, when lying or telling the truth; the attractive appearance of the listener perhaps distorted the non-verbal behavior of the speaker (DePaulo, 1985).

Implications of this study are:

i. A very attractive doctor may make a patient appear insincere (and *vice versa*).
ii. Written history, even through a computer, can mask all the non-verbal cues of truth, sincerity or deception.

To explain how people judge that others are lying, an *expectancy-violation model* has been proposed. According to the model, deception is perceived from non-verbal behavior that violates normative expectation. In studies conducted in USA and in India, people exhibited weird non-verbal behaviors (arm raising, head-tilting, staring, etc.) while speaking. American undergraduates as well as Indian illiterates inferred deception from these weird behaviors. This was consistent with the expectancy-violation model (Bond, 1992). In hospital setting too, this model seems to be operational.

Implications of this study are that weird behavior by a doctor may be inferred as signs of deception by the patients, both literate and illiterate. Sticking to expectant model of behavior in one's dress, appearance and communication enhances his/her credibility. "In Rome, do as Romans do" sums it up well.

True and Deceptive Smiles

Subtle differences among forms of smiling could be distinguished. Muscular activity around the eyes ('smiling with the eyes') along with the smiling lips occurred more often when people were actually enjoying themselves. When a smile was feigned to conceal negative emotions, it included traces of disgust, fear, contempt, or sadness (Ekman, 1988). The message is, "The eyes smile truly while the lips may deceive." So, observe the patients' eyes when they smile.

Chronic Blushing

Severe chronic blushing is associated with social anxiety, anxiety state and depression (Edelmann, 1991). It is common in our young unsophisticated womenfolk, especially teenage girls and unmarried women from rural areas. One should be more tactful and gentle in communicating with them.

Laughter

Laughter is a unique and ubiquitous human phenomenon. Until recently, medical research has neglected laughter and relegated it to philosophers and naturalists, particularly Darwin.

Laughter, as a behavior, has many causes, including humour, incongruity, relief, and a sense of well being. *Laughter may have developed for its cathartic effects and adaptive value.* As an evolutionary device, laughter may have served to thwart aggression, spread information, and preserve social unity. Laughter has a great potential for a variety of clinical uses that awaits further research (Black, 1984).

Laughter and Pain Threshold

Two experiments have been conducted to test the proposal that laughter is a pain antagonist. Discomfort thresholds were higher for subjects in the laughter and the relaxation inducing conditions provide by audiotapes or narratives. Laughter, and not simply distraction, reduces discomfort sensitivity, suggesting that laughter has potential as an intervention strategy for the reduction of clinical discomfort (Cogan, 1987).

Laughter and Stress Hormones

Positive emotional activities have been suggested as modifiers of neuro-endocrine hormones involved in the classical stress response. The mirthful laughter experience of watching a comedy for 60 minutes appears to reduce serum levels of cortisol, dopac, epinephrine, and growth hormone. These biochemical changes indicate reversal of the classical neuro-endocrine and hormone response to stress (Berk, 1989).

Humour as Therapy

Laughter is an effective placebo while fear is a potent *nocebo*. The main effects of therapeutic humour are symptom relief and increased cohesion between a doctor and a patient. Humour may have a therapeutic value when it is associated with the following principles:

i. A positive doctor-patient relationship that includes the *freedom to be humorous*;
ii. The humour used is life affirming and is not cynical or negative;
iii. The humour increases social cohesion;
iv. The humour is interactive;
v. The humour reduces stress.

These principles are not to be applied in an isolated manner. One should combine it with other principles of doctor-patient dyad. One should also be aware when humour is or is not appropriate (Richman, 1995). The movie 'Patch Adams' (1998) highlights some of these principles rather well.

Psychology of Crying

Crying is caused by the ego state getting temporarily inundated by complex memories and feelings. At that moment, the overwhelmed ego cannot provide appropriate and integrated verbal response. Words and verbal thinking fail. The initiating emotion may be one of *sadness, gratitude, love, pride, or joy* (Wood, 1984).

If a patient feels tearful during consultation, it indicates that pleasant or unpleasant thoughts and feelings overwhelm him/her. It is my observation that most patients cry in front of you only when they have adequate rapport with you and do not mind letting their ego state get overwhelmed in your presence. I consider it a good sign of rapport building when a new case cries during the dyad. Empathetic listening helps to control the crying faster and more effectively than sympathy.

Crying and Expression

Study subjects, who cried in response to watching a sad movie, were more expressive and felt more sadness and pain than the subjects who did not cry. Crying also was associated with increases in somatic and autonomic nervous system activity. Crying is thus associated with an aversive state of arousal, that includes negative emotion and a complex mixture of sympathetic, parasympathetic, and somatic activation (Gross, 1994).

The implications are two: 1) Patients, who are known to cry easily, say in movie halls, may feel more pain and express it better to a doctor. 2) Those who cry less are likely to be more stoic and less expressive about their distressing symptoms like aches and pains. A competent doctor may use this to fine-tune a dyad by *coaxing the quiet* or double-checking the severity of symptoms by indirect questioning.

Weeping and Humour on Stress

The moderating effects of emotional weeping and humour on the impact of negative life events were examined in a study. Compared to those who rarely wept, those who wept frequently showed more mood disturbance at high levels of negative events and less to low levels of negative events. Humour buffered stress in all groups except for males who reported frequent crying (Labott, 1987).

This study implies that crying acts as a buffer and helps to cope with minor setbacks in life but not major ones. Laughter, on the contrary, helped in all situations except in *male cry-babies.* In real life dyads, we find that crying and smiling are two sides of a coin. Patients, who shed tears while recounting their distressing experiences, most often smile or laugh later when they feel unburdened by *getting it all off their chest.*

Odour as a Signal

Old textbooks of clinical medicine list several odours indicative of various diseases. In a study, when asked to attach the attributes 'pleasant', 'indifferent' or 'unpleasant' to several odours, the subjects judged female odours more often pleasant and less often unpleasant than male odours (Hold, 1977). Be odourless or wear a pleasant and mild perfume. Patients may perceive it as a non-verbal signal of a pleasant person. At the same time, avoid excessive use of cosmetics; patients may perceive it as a sign of frivolousness.

DOCTOR'S NON-VERBAL SKILLS AND PATIENT SATISFACTION

A doctor's non-verbal behavior may communicate emotion and feelings toward a patient. Thus, skilled utilisation of appropriate non-verbal cues should facilitate therapy.

The three dimensions of non-verbal communication are:

i. *Immediacy* (close distance and eye contact during the dyad),
ii. *Potency* or *status* (seating, palpating, and other privileges that differentiate the doctor) and
iii. *Responsivity* (ability to receive and appropriately respond to a patient's verbal and non-verbal cues).

A study has demonstrated that *immediacy* is the basis for interpretations of empathy, warmth, genuineness, and effectiveness (Sherer, 1980). In another study, patient satisfaction correlated strongly with ratings for physician courtesy and information giving (*responsivity*) but not with non-verbal behaviors of *immediacy* and *potency* (Comstock, 1982).

The relationship between physicians' non-verbal communication skills and their patients' satisfaction with medical care was examined in two other studies. The patients commented on measures of satisfaction with the technical aspects (the 'science') and the socio-emotional aspects (the 'art') of the medical care they received. The non-verbal communication skills of the physicians bore no relationship to patients' ratings of the technical quality of care. However, measures of these skills did predict patient satisfaction with the art of medical care received. Physicians who were more sensitive to body movement and posture cues to emotion, received higher ratings on the art of care than did less sensitive physicians. Thus, patients are able to discriminate between *scientific competence* and *art of practice* shown by doctors.

In addition, physicians who were successful at expressing emotion through their non-verbal communications tended to receive higher ratings from patients on the art of care than did physicians who were less effective communicators (DiMatteo, 1980). Another study by the same researchers demonstrated that physician sensitivity to audio communication predicted patient compliance; physicians, who were more sensitive to patients' verbal output, experienced fewer appointment cancellations (DiMatteo, 1986).

The message seems to be, '*Develop your Emotional Quotient (EQ) to practise artfully and prosper; update your science and skills to impress your patients.*'

Do's and Don'ts to Project a Better Image

1. At all times, listen to the patient's non-verbal signals and respond appropriately.
2. Spoken words should be clear, jargon-free, unhurried and unambiguous.
3. Voice tone should be friendly and reveal concern for the patient by varying appropriately. Most patients can see through mechanically modulating the voice without empathy.
4. Gestures and expressions should be open and friendly. Maintain appropriate eye contact and stay comfortably close according to the gender, age and personality of the patient.
5. Dress, grooming and possessions should reveal that you are a careful and cultured person. Flashy dress and possessions are best avoided while on duty.
6. A physician intending to practice for long in a particular location should develop worthy affiliations and avoid those that may spoil one's image in public eye.

SUMMARY

It must be clear by now that acquiring NVB literacy involves commitment on one's part to perceive the various individual signs and then comprehend the major signals. Acquiring mastery in NVB literacy is a life-long voyage of discovery that is at once challenging and exhilarating. Start on yours today.

BIBLIOGRAPHY

1. Berk LS, Tan SA, Fry WF, Napier BJ, Lee JW, Hubbard RW, Lewis JE, Eby WC. Neuroendocrine and stress hormone changes during mirthful laughter. American Journal of the Medical Sciences. 1989; 298:390-6.
2. Black DW. Laughter. JAMA. 1984;252:2995-8.
3. Bond CF Jr, Omar A, Pitre U, Lashley BR, Skaggs LM, Kirk CT. Fishy looking liars: deception judgment from expectancy violation. Journal of Personality and Social Psychology. 1992;63:969-77.
4. Bond MH, Komai H, Targets of gazing and eye contact during interviews: effect on Japanese nonverbal behavior. Journal of Personality and Social Psychology. 1976;34:1276-84.
5. Chesney MA, Ekman P, Friesen WV, Black GW, Hecker MH. Type A behavior pattern: facial behavior and speech components. Psychosomatic Medicine. 1990; 52:307-19.
6. Cogan R, Cogan D, Waltz W, McCue M. Effects of laughter and relaxation on discomfort thresholds. Journal of Behavioral Medicine. 1987;10:139-44.
7. Comstock LM, Hooper EM, Goodwin JM, Goodwin JS. Physician behaviors that correlate with patient satisfaction. Journal of Medical Education. 1982;57:105-12.
8. Craig KD, Hyde SA, Patrick CJ. Genuine, suppressed and faked facial behavior during exacerbation of chronic low back pain. Pain. 1991;46:161-71.
9. Craig KD, Patrick CJ. Facial expression during induced pain. Journal of Personality and Social Psychology. 1985;48:1080-91.
10. DePaulo BM, Stone JI, Lassiter GD. Telling ingratiating lies: effects of target sex and target attractiveness on verbal and nonverbal deceptive success. Journal of Personality and Social Psychology. 1985;48:1191-203.
11. DiMatteo MR, Hays RD, Prince LM. Relationship of physicians' nonverbal communication skill to patient satisfaction, appointment noncompliance, and physician workload. Health Psychology. 1986;5:581-94.
12. DiMatteo MR, Taranta A, Friedman HS, Prince LM. Predicting patient satisfaction from physicians' nonverbal communication skills. Medical Care. 1980;18:376-87.
13. Edelmann RJ. Correlates of chronic blushing. British Journal of Clinical Psychology. 1991;30:177-8.
14. Ekman P, Friesen WV, O'Sullivan M. Smiles when lying. Journal of Personality and Social Psychology. 1988;54:414-20.
15. Greden JF, Genero N, Price HL. Agitation-increased electromyogram activity in the corrugator muscle region: a possible explanation of the "Omega sign"?. American Journal of Psychiatry. 1985; 142:348-51.
16. Gross JJ. Frederickson BL, Levenson RW. The psychophysiology of crying. Psychophysiology. 1994; 31:460-8.
17. Hold B, Schleidt M. The importance of human odour in nonverbal communication. Zeitschrift fur Tierpsychologie. 1977;43:225-38.
18. Iizuka Y. Extraversion, introversion, and visual interaction. Perceptual and Motor Skills. 1992;74:43-50.
19. Labott SM, Martin RB. The stress moderating effects of weeping and humor. Journal of Human Stress. 1987;13:159-64.

20. Mandal MK, Pandey R, Madan SK. Exposed eye area (EEA) in the expression of various emotions. Journal of General Psychology. 1992;119:385-9.
21. Marcos LR. Nonverbal behavior and thought processing. Archives of General Psychiatry. 1979;36:940-3.
22. Muller D, Chambliss J. Hand, body and viewing behaviors of students with high or low self-concepts. Perceptual and Motor Skills. 1980;50:709-10.
23. Poole GD, Craig KD. Judgments of genuine, suppressed, and faked facial expressions of pain. Journal of Personality and Social Psychology. 1992;63:797-805.
24. Prkachin KM. Dissociating spontaneous and deliberate expressions of pain: signal detection analyses. Pain. 1992;51:57-65.
25. Richman J. The lifesaving function of humor with the depressed and suicidal elderly. Gerontologist. 1995;35:271-3.
26. Searles HF. The role of the analyst's facial expressions in psychoanalysis and psychoanalytic therapy. International Journal of Psychoanalytic Psychotherapy. 1984-85;10:47-73.
27. Sherer M, Rogers RW. Effects of therapists nonverbal communication on rated skill and effectiveness. Journal of Clinical Psychology. 1980;36:696-700.
28. Wagner RE, Hexel M, Bauer WW, Kropiunigg U. Crying in hospitals: a survey of doctors,' nurses' and medical students' experience and attitudes. Medical Journal of Australia. 1997;166:13-6.
29. Weil NH. The role of facial expressions in the holding environment. International Journal of Psychoanalytic Psychotherapy. 1984-85;10:75-89.
30. Wood EC, Wood CD. Tearfulness: a psychoanalytic interpretation. Journal of the American Psychoanalytic Association. 1984;32:117-36.

PRACTICAL EXERCISES

Body Language Training

These exercises are designed to help students tune in to the subtleties of body language.

i. *Hand Gestures*: Ask students to demonstrate and describe the meaning of various hand gestures. You will be amazed at how many there are. Discuss how facial expressions and other body movements that influence the meaning of a hand gesture. What do hand gestures mean in different cultures?

ii. *Body Behavior*: Discuss body language in a ward or lab. What personality types can you detect just by how people use their bodies? What are the obvious and subtle behaviors of the braggart, the flirt, the wallflower, the stoic, etc.? Consider such factors as personal space, posture, eye contact, speed and angle of movement.

iii. *The Mind Reader ("Tell")*: Gamblers and con artists long have known that people reveal their inner thoughts through body language without even knowing it. For example, if you place a coin in one hand behind your back and then present your fists to a body-savvy person, that person may be able to detect where the coin is. Your "tell" will indicate which hand holds it. You may lean your body to one side, hold one hand higher than the other, point your nose, or unintentionally leak some other behavior that gives away your "secret."

Have students form pairs to try this coin experiment. Some people are much more adept at it than others. If you are good at it yourself, demonstrate with a volunteer in front of the class. This exercise works best if the person with the coin is not told (initially) about the concept of the "tell."

iv. *Mirroring*: Have the students pair off. Either sitting or standing, one person in each pair takes the lead and begins to move in any way he/she wishes (tell them to avoid talking, since it is distracting). The task for the other student is to follow or mimic everything that the leader does. Encourage people to use both obvious and subtle behaviors. Do this for a minute or two, then switch roles of who is leading and who is following. Finally, tell the dyads to do the exercise one last time except that *no one* is the leader or the follower. Both people in the pair should try to move in unison, as if they are mirroring each other simultaneously in a body language "dance." This is somewhat hard to do and takes a bit of practice before a pair gets the hang of it, if they can do it at all. If the pair is successful, what usually happens is that there are rapid, minute shifts between leading and following. This mirroring can be done with body language alone, facial expressions alone, or body language with facial expressions. This last one is considerably more difficult to do than the first two.

This simple exercise sensitises the students to the details of body movement and expression. It also may say something about interpersonal styles. Some students prefer to "lead" while others prefer to "follow." In particular, some people are very empathetically in tune with the others movements, while some people cannot focus on this. In addition, moving in unison is easy with some people, but not others.

Role-play

Role-play of major non-verbal signals by student volunteers. The important ones are deception, concealed hostility and disbelief. These signals are common in Indian patients. Non-compliant patients reveal NVB of deception, patients with chronic intractable problems reveal—variably concealed—hostility and any patient, who can not understand '*disease-illness paradox,*' reveals signs of disbelief. One student can play the doctor and three others play three patients who reveal deception, concealed hostility and disbelief respectively. The other student observe the role-plays and then tutor conducts a debriefing during which, the signals picked up and missed could be discussed. If video recording and play back is available, it will be even more effective.

Video Triggers

Brief segments from TV of cinema can be collected to show various components of communication like body language, para-language, possessions, appearance, etc.

Demonstration of Specific Signs

A trained dancer or a drama actor can be invited to demonstrate specific non-verbal cues of the eyes. face, etc.

Observation and Feedback

The students act as assessors of non-verbal cue in live or recorded doctor patient dyads. Their notes are then discussed in a plenary feedback session where the errors of omission and commission are pointed out.

CHAPTER

5

Answering Skills

> *Genius not only diagnoses the situation but supplies the Answers.*
>
> —Robert Graves

INTRODUCTION

This is perhaps one of the weakest communication skill among Indian medical professionals. Though patient load, lack of time, difficulty in explaining hi-tech medical care to an illiterate, etc. are cited as reasons for this state of affairs, the fact remains that most third world patients feel *defensive* while asking questions to doctors. Many of them start a question with an apology. This should not happen if we claim to practise *patient centred* medicine.

In a consumer meet, a prominent city surgeon declared that he was a skilled surgeon and his *only job was to operate well.* He had been trained to take care of only the surgical problems of his patients and it was not his job to please them with his communication skill. The point he had missed and no consumer pointed out to him was that *taking care* of a patient meant *caring for the organs, body and the mind of the patient.* Today, even a robot could be trained to perform a surgical procedure. Being human means being inclusive, holistic and humane. As Peabody reminded us, "*Patient care means to care for the patient.*"

In Indian context, patient satisfaction is largely decided by the quality of answers and explanations given by a doctor. It can cover deficiencies in other aspects of doctor-patient communication. It is also a relatively easy skill to develop, easier than acquiring skills of questioning and listening.

TIPS ON ANSWERING PATIENT'S QUERIES

Listen

Listen carefully; show interest by nodding, smiling, leaning towards the patient, etc. (see 'Positive Signals')

Understand

If the question is not clear, repeat or paraphrase the question and check with the patient if you have understood it correctly.

Elicit Opinion First

To a thought-provoking question, elicit the patient's opinion before giving your answer.

Prepare

Be prepared with your answers. After all you know more about diseases than the patient, though thanks to Internet access, many of them come well prepared with the latest information.

Answer

Answer fully and clearly but briefly. Patients often ask closed-ended questions that could be answered with yes/no.

Be Truthful

Do not bluff an answer if you cannot give a ready answer. Compliment the patient on asking a good question and ask some time to refer and get back. However, this may backfire with patients of traditional type who believe that doctors should know all answers with out referring to books; you may lose their respect. Manage such cases with a noncommittal reply and gain time to refer journals by saying one of the following:

- "Certain tests, the results of which are awaited, would help give a more specific and individualised answer",
- "Your disease in its early stage; we have to watch for some time before I can give you a specific answer" or
- "This is the first time you have consulted me. Let me observe you for some more time before answering that."

Be Honest but not Brutal

When answering questions on management options, be cautiously optimistic; highlight the benefits of therapy in a strong positive way. Do not talk only of the cost and risk but balance it with the benefit. As Needleham put it, "*A brutally honest person enjoys brutality quite as much as honesty; possibly even more*!"

Euphemism in doctors' language: Several medical terms have stigma or negative emotive appeal; doctors overcome this problem by the use of euphemisms, which are neutral and less emotive (e.g. 'retro-V' for HIV, "congested lung" for "heart failure", etc). By such acts, they may protect patients' feelings at the cost of being labelled less open (Tayler M and Ogden J, 2005). At times, the plain English may be more upsetting than the medical term: A study assessed the outcome when doctors avoided the term 'obese' and used an euphemism such as 'your weight may be damaging your health'; the patients felt that the medical term 'obese' made the problem appear more serious but it was less upsetting to them than the euphemism in plain English (Tailor A and Ogden J, 2009).

Similarly, the use of a medical term may facilitate shared decision-making if a patient can understand it correctly. On the other hand, it may be misunderstood. Experiments show that with a medical label (i.e. Tonsillitis), the patients felt that their illness has been taken seriously and had greater confidence in the doctor, while the lay diagnosis (i.e. Sore throat) made the patient feel more ownership of the problem.

Get Feedback

After completing your answer, verify with the patient verbally or by body language that you have given a satisfactory reply. Often we use jargon or say things that a patient can not follow. Feedback ensures that our answer has been understood. The best way of ensuring that your patients have understood is to make them repeat what you have told them. This is especially useful after you give treatment advice to check if they have understood all that you have told them to do.

Going Beyond the Question

Think 'Why?' and 'Why Now?'

Problematic situations occur often during question-answer sessions. One must develop the habit of asking oneself *"Why this question?"* and *"Why now?"* Over a period, one develops the insight required to identify the hidden agenda behind such questioning.

Confusion

Some patients are confused, lost, and may want some clarifications and a lot of support. They blurt out any question that comes to their mind. This is common in medical emergencies. Empathise and reassure them rather than chiding for asking *stupid questions*. Guide them to focus on the problem.

Control

Relatives, especially the dominant spouse or parent, who accompany patients, feel left out whenever the patient is in the spotlight; they often butt in with queries just to regain control. They are interested in the process of questioning and not really in what you answer. Even an acknowledgement from you that you have registered their concern is enough.

Obsession

Some patients, especially the hypochondriacs, are tenacious and will pursue a point relentlessly. Many chronic patients with irritable bowel syndrome, tension headache, chronic pain syndrome, phobias, etc. may literally "drive you nuts" with queries related to their beliefs and idiosyncrasies. You need time and patience to handle them well. If time is a constraint, do not brush them off; give them another appointment for counselling.

Hostility

Some hostile or cynical patients may openly disagree with you and announce so loudly that others can hear (see "Hostile patient").

Disbelief

Some patients may be "habitual disbelievers", who will question all your decisions and suggestions, if it is not already known and acceptable to them. Patients from *the rich and famous* category, priests, teachers and top professionals may belong to this category. I have found that if you can impress them with your expertise and concern for their welfare, they turn out to be your ardent fans (see "Superior personality").

Think 'How?'

Think *how* a question has been framed. The way it is worded gives certain clues. For example, curiosity, suspicion and prejudice could alter the form of a question in the following manner:

Curiosity

"I *wonder* if my BP is high due to poor sleep last night. Is it possible?"

Suspicion

"*Can* my BP be *really* so high? I never had any problems till now."

Prejudice

"I *cannot* have high BP. I am a cool person and no one in my family has it. I do not think it can happen to me."

Hostility

"Now that my BP is high, have you not *found a weapon* to brainwash me and give up all the things I like in life."

Though all the four questions are on high BP, the way they are worded suggest underlying emotional tone in each case. Your answers need to be worded appropriately in each case (see "Personality types").

Talk Effectively and Impress Your Patients

Have you ever wondered how some consultants improvise almost perfectly when giving advice to patients? It is as if they always know exactly what to say and how to say it. They seem to have acquired some secret skill on how to spontaneously provide a cohesive and convincing advice. Cultivating the following presentation skills will help you to achieve such mastery:

1. Show eagerness to share relevant information with the patient. Your words will have passion and seem convincing. Dale Carnegie believed that this was critical to getting attention.
2. Be organised and prepared. Be ready with facts and figures related to the case on hand.
3. Use evidences and research findings to gain attention.
4. Know your patients. Sometimes, it goes beyond medical knowledge. For example, dressing appropriately could impress them. You may choose a more conservative look if attending a geriatric clinic. You might be more casual in front of children. Be professional and tasteful at all times.

5. Relate to your patient with your eyes. The eyes are the windows to the soul. Look at people when you talk. The rule of thumb is to look at the person for at least two to five seconds, every time you speak to him/her.
6. Keep your posture straight and natural. This takes a lot of practice, especially when talking about delicate matters. The result is total confidence and control (see "Confidence signals").
7. Vary your voice pattern. Use pauses to make a point.
8. Be aware of your hands and gestures. Your body is the number one visual aid. Practice in front of a mirror or ask your peers to watch your expressions and gestures and give a feedback. Otherwise, you may end up like a professor of surgery, who used to gesture a large incision all along his torso, while trying to reassure his patients that the proposed surgery was only minor!
9. Be animated while being yourself. Develop your own style. Although it is great to emulate other role models, just be your natural self.
10. Learn how to answer questions and objections. Do it in a non-defensive way. Have a positive feeling about what you present. Project to you patient what s/he wants to hear, viz., "What is in it for the patient?" and "How will it affect him/her?"

Have One Theme at a Time

The mind can take in only so much information at one time. Make sure not to give your patient information overload. Develop a structure with up to five main points and back up the points with support that revolves around one central theme at a time like "treatment options in your case".

Use Simple, Action-oriented Language

Simple does not mean elementary. Do not baby talk unless you are addressing a baby! What you do is to make it easy for the patient to understand and digest. Keep your talk 'E-A-S-Y':

- E - Enthusiasm and energy are the keys. Be lively and reactive when you talk with a patient.
- A - Articulate your message. Clarity is essential.
- S - Simple, short and to the point. Use the *KISS principle*: 'Keep it short and simple'.
- Y - Your audience (patients and their relatives): focus on them.

Convey the Right Conceptual Quantity

Do you remember some of your teachers who are big thinkers? They think and talk in holistic, global and abstract terms about "the big picture" and "the whole story." Their statements are often ambiguous and non-specific. You have probably also experienced some detail-oriented teachers who will not be satisfied unless they conveyed all the minute details to you. Similarly, your patients also vary in their ability to handle information; some can take only generalities while others may need details.

Talking in small, details to "global thinkers" will not build rapport. They cannot perceive or process details of that minuscule size. For example, when I talk to such a patient about details of prognosis, s/he would interrupt and ask, "Doctor, is it *Good of Bad*?" In contrast, a detail-oriented patient will not be satisfied with such general comments and may ask, "Doctor, good outlook means what?" and continue to seek clarification on details.

Try to match the size of the facts and concepts in your answers to the patient's capacity to handle details. Listen and estimate their *conceptual chunk* capacity. When you are able to match them, you will be understood well.

End with Emotional Appeal

Appeal to what matters most—hope, health and quality of life. Paint a verbal picture that your audience can grasp. Empathise and take a position of 'realistic optimism.' Keep in mind, *it is not always what you say, but how you say it.*

ADVANCED SKILLS

Answering Objections

In modern day practice, many patients who consult you may have objections to your advice and suggestions. These may be openly stated by the bolder or educated patients while the meek or illiterate ones may only reveal through non-verbal signals. If there were no objections to be raised and clarifications to be sought, then any robot can treat patients to their satisfaction. An objection is therefore both a challenge and an opportunity to show your mettle. Welcome objections and not dread them. After all, it is through those objections you learn your patient's needs and wants, dislikes and fears—in fact, everything you need to know in order to plan an effective, appropriate and acceptable management plan. It is critical that all health professionals learn how to handle objections effectively.

Here are some strategies to make your patient's objections work for you rather than against you:

See the Objection as a Question

If you see the objection as an attack, the natural tendency will be to defend yourself. This promotes an attacker/defender relationship rather than a fiduciary one in which you gain respect and trust. However, if you mentally change the objection into a question, you can proceed to explain to the patient. This would bring back the doctor/patient relationship to its care provider/care seeker mode. For example, if a patient objects to surgical option advised by you, do not get upset. Convert his objection into questions like, "Why do you object? May I know?"

Turn the Objection into a Reason for Following Your Advice

If you can show the patient that whatever the objection is, it is actually the reason to follow your suggestion, you will effectively defuse the objection.

For example, many elderly patients, when advised some surgical procedure, say hernia-repair, will immediately object and say, "No doctor, no surgery for me! I am too old for that." or words to that effect. Pause for a few moments, ponder over his objection and then tell him, "That is precisely why I advice elective surgery now. You are getting older and hernias generally grow bigger with time. Finally, when you agree for surgery to be done, the surgeon may tell you that you are too old to be operated as a low risk case." (see "Mental Judo")

Smoke Out all the Important Objections

If you feel the patient has some reason for not following your line of thinking, simply ask him/her what it is. After he tells you, you verify if that is his only objection. If he says "No," you continue asking, "What else?" until all the objections are out in the open. If s/he says that the objection you have uncovered is the only one, you then ask if you were to eliminate the objection would s/he agree to follow your advice. In order to continue, you need a "Yes" answer to this question. Once you have a definite yes, the patient is committed to accepting your advice if you successfully eliminate his objection. Now you can focus your mind on this single point, and once you clear it up, you would have successfully convinced the patient. In the example cited above, if 'old age' is the only objection to accepting surgical option, then if you convince him that his age is not 'old enough' to rule out safe-surgery, he will have no other reason to refuse surgery.

Admitting to the Objection

When a patient objects to a real limitation, for example, "The procedure you suggest is risky," it is better to admit it. Having done that, continue your presentation focusing on the benefits of following your advice. However, if you try to convince the patient that something is safe when it is obviously not, you will antagonise him especially if there is an adverse outcome after following your advice. Most of the litigation raised by the patients is due to misunderstanding of risk-benefit or cost-benefit of treatment options. It is prudent not to gloss over high-risk and highly expensive procedures.

Let the Patient Answer His Own Objection

If a patient cannot answer your question, "Why do you say so?" then he has disproved himself. The patient may flounder around a bit and then admit his objection was not important. This is especially useful on general objections such as, "I cannot find the time to do exercises."

Agree with the Patient about Something

Find some point of agreement with your patient before you start to answer an objection. This is the best-known way to cushion your answer and render it unobjectionable. The patient will not object as much if he knows that you understand his problem. Mirroring body postures is one easy way of showing agreement by body language.

Repeat the Objection in Your Own Words Before Answering

Repeating the objection serves three purposes:

i. It lets the patient know that you are listening to him.
ii. It helps avoid misunderstandings and ensures that you answer the right question.
iii. It gives you a little time to think about how you are going to reply.

Eliminate Objections with Probing Questions

If you try to overcome objections by arguing with the patients, you may win the argument but lose the patient. In fact this is quite common in government hospitals due to the "Take it or leave it" attitude prevalent there.

You need not overwhelm the objection by sound arguments; you eliminate it through questions at the beginning of the presentation. The initial questioning phase of the consultation is usually pretty relaxed and allows you to find out a great deal about your patient before s/he becomes defensive. If the patient tells you that s/he is the decision-maker, for example, and does not have to check with anyone else, s/he cannot use this as an excuse later not to take a decision on his/her treatment. Many common objections can be eliminated with the proper use of probing questions. (see 'Probing questions').

Deny the Objection

If the objection is obviously untrue, you can smile and say, "Of course I do not believe that." For reasons known only to them, some patients will test you with some outlandish objections. If you try to logically answer illogical objections, you will be sucked into a long, drawn-out and usually fruitless ordeal. Show the patient that you have all your cards on the table and expect him to do the same (see "Why do not you? Yes-but" game).

Get into the Right Mental Attitude and Stay in it

You know you are trying to persuade the patient to accept something s/he needs, something that will benefit him/her but something s/he may dislike and not want. Such *needs versus wants* mismatches are ubiquitous. You are there to render a professional service. If the patient raises a string of objections, do not be upset. If you seem upset, it only reinforces the patient's fears that made him/her raise those objections. More over, getting upset and saying, "It is your health that is at stake—take it or leave it" may be all right for a vendor but not a true professional.

In addition, your body language, appearance, posture and manner of speech must all express confidence and high self-esteem. The way your patient perceives your service is closely tied to how s/he perceives you.

Responding to Disagreements

Even after your best effort, at times your patients may continue to disagree with your advice. Here are some strategies to deal with it.

Tackle the Big Picture First

Disagreement is more often in the details, where specifics can be mismatched or unacceptable to the patient. For example, a long-standing diabetic with proximal muscle weakness due to amyotrophy refused to take insulin injections. He had 'needle-phobia' since childhood. Arguing about the 'painless pricks' did not work with him. One had to make him understand that diabetic amyotrophy was a sign of poor control; unless he achieved a good control of sugar, the muscle weakness would remain and he may be confined to a wheel chair for life. The big picture (Your choice—Insulin or Wheel chair?) when supported by evidence and proof, might be accepted by the patient.

Agree on the Higher Purpose First

Once there is agreement on the big picture, it is easy to talk about higher purpose of treatment. Higher purpose ideas are difficult to disagree with, because they are less specific and vague.

In the preceding example of the case of diabetic amyotrophy, one can strive for a general agreement on the utmost need to get the patient back on his feet at the earliest. Most patients will find it impossible to disagree on this point. Once this is achieved, then details could be worked out. I even let some patients to try unproven therapies to let them discover the hard way that they have to accept professional advice and agree for insulin injections, if they wanted to recover and walk home. In fact, I tell them to try insulin for 'my sake' and if they did not improve within six to eight weeks, I myself would ask them to stop taking the injections. It has always worked. Once the initial resistance is overcome, it is easier to coax them to continue with the therapy.

In short, the strategy and methods are:

i. Agree on the higher purpose of case management first.
ii. Negotiate the required (lower level) detail.
iii. If deadlocked in disagreement, return to higher level and restate the agreed higher purpose.
iv. Negotiate the required detail along alternate paths (see "Negotiating Skills").

Conveying Commitment (*4+ Yes*)

It is not enough to be committed to quality patient care; you should be able to convey it to your patients effectively. You need to realise how an affirmative answer can vary from mild to strong in its effect on the listener. Then you will be able to match the strength of your affirmation to the strength of your commitment.

Imagine that you are speaking with one of your friends. When you ask him, "Shall we get together after work tomorrow, maybe shop and look around?" he replies in four different ways:

1. *Your friend says, "Hmmm."*
   What are the odds that your friend will actually meet you after work tomorrow? It is not good. Technically, the response of "Hmmm" means, "Yes." However, in practice, it can mean—
   a. Yes
   b. A qualified yes—"I have to think about it."
   c. "No, but I do not want to get into it right now."
   d. "I am *not* paying attention to what you are saying; it is just an automatic response that requires no thought."

   Since everyone knows "hmmm" is a very feeble yes at best, we seldom believe it when we hear it. We can give it 1 plus (+) in terms of *yes value.*
2. *Your friend says—"yes, sure" or "fine."*
   "Yes" or words like "sure" are generally perceived as stronger than "hmmm". They are less likely to be used automatically. Still, they lack real conviction. Your friend is definitely saying yes, but what are the odds that answer will change to no by tomorrow afternoon? We can give "yes", "sure", and most other one-word yes responses 2-plus (++) value.
3. *Your friend says, "Definitely, I would like that" or "Absolutely, I have been wanting to get together with you, too."*
   In this case, there is no question your friend was listening to you, and that the response is a solid yes. Your friend demonstrated a strong yes in two ways. He used a very enthusiastic yes word, such as definitely, absolutely or great and said yes in more than one way. We can give multiple, enthusiastic yes 3-plus (+++) value.

4. *Your friend says, "Great, I have been wanting to call you myself. Tell you what. The ward rounds should be over about 4:30. I need another 30 minutes or so to wash up. So let us meet at your place right around 5:00, and then we can go out together."*

What are the odds he will actually meet with you? They could not be higher. Barring an unforeseen problem, your friend will be there. This is a 4-plus (++++) yes. What makes it so are two things, viz, i. the use of enthusiastic yes words to confirm agreement with you and ii. adding and amplifying on what to do to make sure you both meet. Amplification also increases the other person's investment in the outcome. They will try harder to make sure the agreed-to thing will happen, even if a problem does come up.

Using 4-plus Yes in Patient Care

All yes's are therefore not equal. Now let us apply this principle to a common patient care situation:

Patient: *I really need to be operated within a week so that I could join duty next month. Doctor, are you sure you can do it on time?*

Reply 1: *Hmmm.*

Reply 2: *Yes, of course.*

Reply 3: *Positively, I know you must rejoin duty.*

Reply 4: *I am certain we will make that date with time to spare. To make sure, I will personally enter your name in the surgery register and ensure that there are no delays or cancellations. I will confirm your admission date tomorrow.*

Four-plus yes takes more work. In an ideal world where people mean what they say, it should not be necessary. However, they are necessary because most people do not really mean what they say unless they spell out their commitment in detail.

There is one more level beyond the *4+ yes* and that is delivering on your promises time-after time, so the patients learn that when you say, "Yes," you really mean it. It is a 5-plus yes.

Section 1

SUMMARY

Listening, questioning and answering are the three basic activities of doctor-patient dyad. Systematic training and practice will help one master these skills.

BIBLIOGRAPY

1. Several articles on "Answering Skills" in www.salesdoctor.com.
2. Tailor A, Ogden J. Avoiding the term 'obesity': An experimental study of the impact of doctors' language on patients' beliefs. Patient Education and Counseling 2009;76:260-64.
3. Tayler M, Ogden J. Doctors' use of euphemisms and their impact on patients' beliefs about health: An experimental study of heart failure. Patient Education and Counseling 2005;57:321-6.

EXERCISES

Simulation Role-play

Doctor's Answering Skills

Students pair off. Clinical situations are assigned to each pair. These should relate to common occurrences in clinical practice. The 'doctor' talks with the 'patient' who keeps track of the answers given by the doctor and the mode of delivery. (A third student may play the role of 'observer' to note the details of the dyad). In the plenary session, the tutor can discuss the observed errors and guide improvement in answering skills. If video recording is available, feedback session can be more objective.

Skills in Conveying Affirmation

In this role-play, the 'patient' expects an affirmation from the 'doctor.' The strength of affirmation is graded from + to ++++ as per the coding of 'Yes-strength' discussed above. The audience comments on the appropriateness of the affirmation in the context of the disease, outlook and patient expectation. The message is "Affirm *as strongly as needed but not more than what is prudent.*"

Skills in Answering Objections and Disagreements

This may be suitable for interns and PG students or for practising professionals. Devise common scenes of arguments, disagreements and objections from patients (donating blood, undergoing an invasive procedure, not getting the expected prescription, having to take a painful injection are some examples). The role players enact the scene and the audience comment upon the appropriateness.

CHAPTER

6

Information Sharing: Models and Methods

We must learn our limits. We are all something, but none of us are everything.
—Blaise Pascal

INTRODUCTION

The word doctor (*docteur*) means, "to teach." Health professionals need to share information and educate their patients. There is no single best method to do this. Depending on the patient characteristics and the clinical context, different methods may be appropriate. The more important models and methods are discussed in this chapter.

COMMUNICATION PATTERNS IN DOCTOR–PATIENT DYADS

Five distinct communication patterns are identifiable in primary care dyads:

i. Narrowly biomedical—characterised by closed-ended medical questions and biomedical talk.
ii. Expanded biomedical—with limited psychosocial discussion related to biomedical sphere.
iii. Bio-psychosocial—reflecting a balance of psychosocial and biomedical topics.
iv. Psychosocial—characterised by psychosocial exchange.
v. Consumerist—characterised by the patient seeking information and the physician providing it.

A recent study revealed that patient satisfaction was highest in the psychosocial pattern. Physician satisfaction was highest in the consumerist pattern and lowest in the narrowly biomedical pattern. Younger male physicians used narrow biomedically focused pattern more often (Roter, 1997).

MODELS FOR INFORMATION EXCHANGE

Tablel 6.1 highlights the models of information exchange and the roles played by doctor and the patient there in.

Table 6.1: The roles played by doctors and patients in decision-making models

Decision-making model	*Doctors' role*	*Patients' role*
Paternalistic model	Active decision making	Passive and submissive
Informed decision model	Passive source of information	Active decision making
Partnership model	Active decision making by consensus	Active decision making by consensus
Guidance co-operation model	Active decision making	Active co-operation

Paternalistic Model

The characteristics of the paternalistic model are easily surmised. In the purest form of this model, a passive, uninformed patient surrenders to professional competence and authority of the doctor who chooses "the best possible option" for the patient. This model presumes that the doctor will make the best decisions for the patient and can do so without involving him or her in the decision-making process. There is no disclosure, i.e. sharing of any of the decision-making steps in this model. Therefore, by definition, a doctor-patient partnership does not exist.

In cases where both the patient and the doctor prefer this approach, it may be argued that they have entered in to this form of relationship based on mutual agreement. However, the patient may not be aware of other decision-making models and therefore, may think that medical decisions are all made paternalistically. The onus is on the doctor to discuss patients' preferences and take them along the decision-making process.

Even when you ask patients for their preferences, a trusting patient usually replies, "You are the doctor; you have to tell me." This should not be used as a license to adopt the paternalistic model but as a sign that the patient needs your expertise to make the best decision. You have to coax the patient to talk about his/her hope and expectations, and then counsel or guide them to decision-making.

A recent study focussed on the ethical load of being paternalistic (Gafni, 1998). Whenever a patient accepts paternalistic role by a doctor, s/he assumes his/her physician to be a 'perfect agent' for the patient to solve his/her health problems. Being a 'perfect agent' of health care delivery carries two ethical obligations:

- Living up to the image by having *fiduciary relationship* with the patient.
- Educating the patient without inculcating personal bias.

An ethical professional may find playing the paternalistic role of a perfect agent may be much more difficult than other roles in the models discussed below.

Partnership Model

This model assumes that both the patient and the doctor have a legitimate concern in the management decision. The partnership model is interactive in nature; the doctor and patient are *partners* who share responsibility in all stages of the decision-making process. There is a two-way exchange of information between the doctor and the patient on treatment preferences. They agree on the management options to implement by consensus. The challenge for doctors using this model is to create an environment in which the patient feels comfortable expressing his/her treatment preferences, which may include 'doing nothing' or 'watchful expectancy' or 'alternate therapies.'

Informed Decision Model

The informed model is based on a clear division of responsibilities between a patient and the doctor. In the information exchange stage, the doctor leads and the communication is mainly from the doctor to the patient. The doctor informs the patient on all relevant treatment options and their benefits and risks. The patient makes an informed treatment decision. This corresponds to the "consumerist" pattern of dyads.

This model assumes that the patient is solely responsible for contemplation and decision-making. Information transfer is seen as the only legitimate contribution of the doctor in making the decision. The doctor is accorded no legitimate claim for involvement in actual decision making. This model believes that the people whose preferences matter are the patients, because they are the ones who will have to live (or die) with the outcomes.

This mode may work well with decisions regarding elective and optional procedures like cosmetic surgery where client's choice is of paramount importance. In complex situations, where decision making needs professional insight, uncritical use of this model may be detrimental to patients. Average Indian patients, provided they trust the doctor, do not prefer this model. Making a 'life and death decision' is not the same as buying consumables from a vendor and the patients are usually grateful if their doctor shares the responsibility of making decisions.

Intermediate Approaches

In addition to the three models, there are other intermediate or hybrid approaches to sharing information and decision-making. *Guidance co-operation model* is quite prevalent in India. In this approach, the doctor actively informs, suggests, and advises and the patient co-operates fully with the doctor in complying with therapy.

In a clinical dyad, the doctor may not use a pure model, but a hybrid of elements of more than one model based on the situation, complexity and patient characteristics. Given the dynamic, complex, and personal nature of the doctor-patient relationship, the decision-making model adopted at the outset of a clinical dyad may be modified to reflect the needs of individual patients.

CLINICAL CONTEXT FOR DOCTOR-PATIENT RELATIONSHIP

When patients consult you for a minor problem (such as common cold) that needs a simple treatment, there is no need to elicit patients' preferences about decision-making, especially in ambulatory care, where the time for each dyad is limited.

The need for some form of shared decision-making is most compelling when the patient presents with a life threatening illness, when different management options exist with varying costs, benefits and risks, and when outcome is unpredictable. In these situations, the stakes are high and there is no single "best" option. The patient will have to bear the consequences of whatever decision is taken and therefore, it is important that his/her preferences are elicited and given their due. Patients in such crises feel vulnerable and may not initiate discussion on management options; *it is the doctor's responsibility to ensure that this occurs and that their views are taken seriously.*

Both time and funding constraints in the current healthcare scene act as disincentives for doctors to elicit patients' preferences while making management decisions. However, *partnership approach* is worth practising as it not only increases patient satisfaction but also reduces the chances of litigation if any adverse outcome results.

Impact of Gender Dyads on Doctor–Patient Communication

Studies (Sandhu et al, 2009) have shown that "Male talk" is predominantly task-orientated; men are more likely to communicate in ways which are louder, more forceful, dominant, and competitive; they interrupt others more frequently. "Female talk" is more likely to be emotional, subjective, polite, and self-revealing; to show more concern and awareness of the feelings of others. Women express and interpret emotions through non-verbal cues more accurately than men. *Remember that a male doctor can adopt 'female talk' and a female doctor can adopt 'male talk.'*

Scientific observations suggest that female doctors involve patients in decision-making and gather information about psychosocial issues more than their male colleagues. Although they offer a more empathetic communication style and spend longer with patients, female doctors make more referrals to hospitals compared with male doctors, and are less cost-effective. This has to be balanced with the patient-centred consulting styles of female doctors leading to better patient outcomes. Compared with female doctors, male doctors are more likely to control consultations, to use medical jargon and to focus more on medical conditions.

Patient gender influences the dyadic process as well: compared with male patients, female patients ask more questions, present more symptoms, give more detailed histories, and get more information with less medical jargon.

PATIENT RELATED VARIABLES

Disclosure of information cannot be uniformly adopted because such disclosures have widely varying effects. Two major patient-related factors are coping style and educational sophistication. Patients, who are highly educated and who follow coping strategies based on active problem solving tend to appreciate the disclosures; they become active partners in decision-making and such involvement reduces their anxiety. They need to know *what, why* and *how* medical decisions are being made.

On the other hand, illiterate patients, who follow passive emotion-focussed coping styles, tend to become more anxious if forced to take part in decision-making. This is our common experience in Government hospitals where rural and rustic patients predominate. Even in this group, the anxiety level reduces if suitable information is given. They need information on *what* is being done and not on *why* or *how* it is going to be done. The Table 6.2 summarises the characteristics of disclosure and non-disclosure models. You can use either of them depending on the clinical context.

Table 6.2: Comparison of disclosure and non-disclosure models

Practice parameters	*Non-disclosure*	*Disclosure*
Dominant culture	Oriental, socially embedded	Western, individual autonomy
Doctor-Patient relationship	Paternalistic, fiduciary	Autonomous patient; doctor as a counsellor
Ideal patient	Trusts with Child-like implicit faith	Informed, empowered to seek clarifications, open, bold
Ideal doctor	Fiduciary "perfect agent"	Friendly "professional partner"
Basis of trust in doctor	Charisma, reputation, personal faith based on experience	Skill, scientific knowledge, honesty and openness
Opinion on information sharing	May kill hope; cruel and unnecessary; "doctor knows best"	Right to know and plan, "knowledge is power"
Style of communication	Indirect, implicit, euphemistic	Direct, explicit, matter of fact
Awareness of patient's disease	Doctor (and family members)	Doctor and patient
Decision makers	Doctor (and family members)	Patient or patient and doctor
Coping behaviour of patients	Accepting, accommodating, emotion-focussed, passive	Challenging, problem solving, solution-focussed, active
Basis of patient's hope	God, fate, passively uncertain	Will-power, science and technology, experimental therapy
Risk taking behaviour	Little; avoids beneficial options if risky	Much more; accepts risky options if beneficial
A "good" death	Unaware, serene, quick; not to be openly discussed with family; Living will unacceptable	Prepared, aware, self-determined, openly discussed with near and dear. Prefers to write a living will to indicate mode of death

THE "PATIENT-PHYSICIAN MATCH" FOR SHARING OF INFORMATION

It is clear from the table above that not all patients prefer patient-centred communication. About 30% prefer the doctor to be their advocates and make management decisions on their behalf. It is therefore necessary for a doctor to assess how much of "Control" each patient wishes to have over his/her healthcare and how "facile" the person is in handling the medical information relevant to the case management (Kiesler et al, 2006).

Based on 'patient control' (low/high) and 'patient's facility' (low/high), there are four possibilities:

Patients with Low Control and Low Facility

Medically unsophisticated, often illiterate, passive recipients of medical information, who depend on their doctor to tell them what to do.

Physician style: Paternalism is appropriate here. "Doctor knows best" role is played out. Inform such patients only the most essential medical information in a very simplified manner.

Patients with Low Control and High Facility

Medically unsophisticated, often dependent personality type, who trusts doctors to be "perfect angels" and comfortable getting advice from them. Wants to know and can digest medical information.
Physician style: Deferential approach is appropriate for such patients. Doctor makes decisions for the patients and discussed fully the medical problems and the management solutions advised.

Patients with High Control and Low Facility

Medically unsophisticated and can not process medical information well, but accustomed to making all decisions and wishes to make medical decisions as well. At times suspicious of doctors intentions.
Physician style: Be a "benign coach" directing and taking the patient along; narrow down the management options to medically sound alternatives and present them in a very simplified manner; present in a way that steers the patient away from making irrational choices. Make the patient feel he/she has made the decision and commit to it.

Patients with High Control and High Facility

Well educated, or well informed and sophisticated; consumerist approach to healthcare; takes an active role in digesting detailed medical information and making decisions, at times after challenging the doctor's opinion.
Physician style: Collaborative participatory approach is best way of dealing with such patients. Emphasise on joint decision making and supply all the relevant medical information and options. Let the patient make the decision and commit to it.

In all the above instances, appropriate emotional and informational support given by the doctor will foster trust between patient and physician.

CO-PRODUCTION OF CONTENT DURING DOCTOR–PATIENT DYAD

Until recently, most studies limited their outlook to the doctors' human interaction skills such as asking for patient opinion, avoiding interruptions, etc. However, the content is as important as the process of information exchange. Collaborative discussion about treatment involves "co-production of content" and refers to the contribution by the doctor and the patient to content generated during the consultation (Richard et al, 2007). An example of the details of content matter discussed during a doctor-patient consultation dyad on drug treatment is listed below:

Drug Guidance-counselling

Content theme categories and specifics

Drug Designation

Medication named
Form of medication
Class named (as a lay person can understand)

Instructions

Instructions for medication (dosage instructions)
Timeframe for expected effect
Duration of treatment
Cost of treatment (especially if patient has to pay for it)
Adjustment of dosage/instructions (if already taken by the patient)
Opinion on strength of medication

Possible Main Effects

Expected effects on symptoms
Action of medication (aligned with the patient's expressed wish to understand)
Observed main effect (if already taken by the patient)
Control of problem
Observed effects on symptoms

Possible Adverse Effect

Possible adverse effects of medication
Precautions against possible adverse effects of medication
Seriousness of possible adverse effects of medication
Probability of possible adverse effects of medication
Observed adverse effect (if already taken by the patient)
Seriousness of observed adverse effects of medication
Precautions (if any) against observed adverse effects of medication
Probability of other adverse effects of medication
Advice on medication (to continue the same or change it)

Warnings

Contraindications of medication
Drug interactions
Allergies/intolerance to medications

Adherence

Elicit patient's commitment to take medication
Check adherence with medication (if already taken by the patient)
Consequences of non-adherence
Solutions for non-adherence

Patient's Attitudes/Emotions

Expression of attitude towards medication and guidance/counselling
Expression of objections regarding medication and guidance/counselling
Expression of doubt about effect of medication and guidance/counselling
Expression of concern regarding medication and guidance/counselling

Indications to return for review and closure

PROACTIVE INFORMATION SHARING: AN EXAMPLE

When patients present with bacterial laryngopharyngitis, a short course of appropriate antibiotic will take care of the infection. However, irritating cough and voice changes may persist leading the patients to continue taking antibiotics or keep consulting various doctors. It is prudent to be proactive in such cases. During the first consultation, they should be informed that while the drugs can cure the *infection*, the *inflammation* will take up to 3 weeks to subside and they should follow non-drug therapy like voice rest, avoidance of ice-cold drinks, etc.

A similar principle works well in cases of minor viral illness. *Proactive information sharing is the key.* If a patient with viral rhinitis, seems to expect an antibiotic, tell them that giving antibiotics prematurely only causes resistant 'bugs' to infect the throat. Treating the 'super bugs' is more difficult and expensive. It is better to wait for 4 to 6 days and watch for signs of secondary bacterial infection—the patient has to look for fever higher than 38.5° C, any change to purulent sputum, foul smelling thick nasal discharge—and report for change in therapy only if needed. This sort of empowerment gives a sense of control to the patients and most of them manage without antibiotics. All this may take a couple of minutes during a dyad but if one wants to practice quality care, it is worth it to spend the extra time than shooting off a prescription for an unnecessary antibiotic (see 'Talking with parents').

Providing other Information Materials

If patients are to be active participants in making healthcare decisions, they need to be given evidence-based information. It should be presented in a form that is acceptable and useful. While information materials are no substitute for good verbal discussions, consultations are usually short and patients may not receive all the information they want and need. Leaflets and other materials can therefore play an important part in supplementing and reinforcing information provided by clinicians, if that information is scientifically accurate, easy to comprehend and relevant.

The growth and wider availability of the Internet will greatly increase access to health information. A Google-search for the term 'health information; yielded about 784,000,000 results in September 2010 and in 21st century, almost all Internet users access the web to retrieve health and medical information. Unfortunately, much of this material is inaccurate or misleading, but it is difficult for non-specialists to sort out the wheat from the chaff. If you could choose a few quality sites of relevance to your patients, they will be glad to empower themselves with appropriate knowledge.

SUMMARY

- Patients' expectations are seldom explicit, and satisfaction is not necessarily related to receiving a great amount of information. Reassurance is often more important and a crucial clinical task.
- Typical methods of imparting reassurance, including allaying fear and anxiety by emphasising the minor or early nature of a disease may not reassure the patients.
- Patients make sense of the doctor's words within the context of their own views and experiences. Therefore, acknowledgement of patients' views of their condition is important for reassurance.

- Consulting techniques that elicit patient expectations, preserve relationships, and facilitate acceptable management options are important.
- Patients who are not acutely ill offer us opportunities to empower them and emphasise positive aspects of rational management.
- The "chagrin" factor (the feeling that your current decision may be seen poorly by hindsight) should be loaded against the unnecessary intervention than for it. Risks to individuals from unnecessary interventions should be emphasised. "One can always intervene later when enough evidence of a disease is apparent. Let me review your condition tomorrow." may work with many patients with self-limiting illnesses.

BIBLIOGRAPHY

1. Butler CC, Rollnick S, Pill R, Maggs-Rapport F, Stott N. Understanding the culture of prescribing: qualitative study of general practitioners' and patients' preceptions of antibiotics for sore throat. BMJ. 1998;317:637-42.
2. Charles C, Gafni A, Whelan T. Decision-making in the physician-patient encounter: Revisiting the shared treatment decision-making model. Soc Sci Med. 1999;49:651-61.
3. Feinstein A. The 'Chagrin Factor' and Qualitative Decision Analysis. Arch Intern Med. 1985;145: 1257-9.
4. Gafni A, Charles C, and Whelan T. The physician-patient encounter: The physician as a perfect agent. Soc. Sci. Med. 1998;47:347-54.
5. Kiesler DJ, Auerbach SM. Optimal matches of patient preferences for information, decision-making and interpersonal behavior: Evidence, models and interventions. Patient Education and Counseling 2006;61:319-41.
6. Margalith I. Shapiro A. Anxiety and Patient participation in Decision-making. Soc Sci Med. 1997;45:419-28.
7. Pauker S, Kassirer J. The threshold approach to clinical decision-making. NEJM. 1980;302(20): 1109-17.
8. Richard C, Lussier MT. Measuring patient and physician participation in exchanges on medications: Dialogue Ratio, Preponderance of Initiative, and Dialogical Roles. Patient Education and Counseling 2007;65:329-41.
9. Roter DL, et al. Communication patterns of primary care physicians. JAMA. 1997;277(4):350-6.
10. Sandhu H, Adams A, Singleton L, Clark-Carter D, Kidd J. The impact of gender dyads on doctor-patient communication: A systematic review. Patient Education and Counseling 2009;76:348-55.

PRACTICAL EXERCISES

1. *Video triggered discussion*: Short doctor-patient dyads can be collected from "medical scenes" in films. The type of information exchange and its appropriateness can be discussed under guidance of an experienced clinician.
2. *Role-playing* is to be done by students on different types of information exchange. A rustic patient, who is comfortable with a paternalistic doctor, a college professor who seeks informed decision-making and a businessperson, who opts for a partnership model are some examples.
3. *Drug advice practice sessions:* Sharing drug information is one of the weak skills of doctors. Using "drug guidance-counselling" checklist given above, a detailed feedback can be given on students practising drug advice with simulated patients (if subject experts act as simulated patients, they can give the feedback on the dyadic process and the content).

CHAPTER

7

Rapport Building Skills

A person attempting to understand life by merely using his reason is like a man trying to take hold of a Flame with the tongs.

—André Gide

INTRODUCTION

Patients' trust in their physicians has recently become a focus of concern, owing largely to the rise of commercialisation of care. Seven categories of physician behaviour that promotes trust were identified in a recent study (Thom, 1997). Only two of them belong to technical competence, viz. thoroughness in evaluation and providing appropriate and effective treatment. The other five belong to interpersonal skills, viz. *understanding patient's individual experience, expressing caring, communicating clearly and completely, building partnership and treating patients with integrity and respect.* The study validated the importance of interpersonal skills in promoting trust.

INTEGRITY AND PATIENT RAPPORT

With the general lack of integrity rampant in the world today, everyone's words seem suspect, including the words of a doctor or a nurse. There is only one reliable way for each of us to counteract the current scepticism. It requires us to demonstrate integrity on a consistent basis while dealing with patients.

- It means promising realistically and delivering more
- It means keeping up your word, regardless of the cost to you
- It means making your word your bond of trust and sincerity.

If you can do all this as a matter of habit, then integrity will be an integral part your dealings with patients.

Ten Ways to Demonstrate Integrity

It is not enough to be a person with integrity; you should be perceived to be so by your patients. For them, perception is reality. Here are ten ways to convey to your patients that you are a professional with integrity.

1. Integrity means adherence to a code of values—sincerity, honesty and candour. Imbibe the meaning of integrity. When you make a statement or promise, stick by it. Make your word your bond of trust and fiduciary relationship with your patients. (See '4+ yes' in chapter 5)
2. Make integrity both a written and unwritten code. Refuse to tolerate false promises from the people you work with. Let it be known that integrity in all your dealings is both expected and delivered.
3. Maintain the same level of integrity in your personal life. (Self test: *If your spouse behaved the way you do when you are away from home, would you be happy with your spouse's behaviour?*)
4. Professionals who make false promises that cannot be fulfilled deserve to lose their practice. Before you commit to a patient, make sure you can honour that commitment. Do not make promises that cannot be fulfilled. They may backfire badly if things go wrong.
5. Use understatement rather than overstatement when committing to a patient. Tell patients what you cannot do; then what you are able to do. For example: "Considering the various risks involved, we may not be able to perform a totally trouble-free surgery, but if trouble does arise, I shall personally provide corrective measures as and when needed."
6. Look people straight in the eye when you make promises. If you feel uncomfortable doing that, you probably will not honour your commitment. Non-verbal signals give away false promises and broken commitments long before they are actually broken.
7. Commit a lot and deliver more. Tell a patient that his recovery may take up to a week, yet discharge him in four days, than promise recovery in four days and keep him for a week. Do not paint yourself into a corner. Make everything you have committed to, happen and then give an extra effort to do even better. Extra efforts are always noticed.
8. Record down your commitments. Make note of each conversation where follow-through or personal effort is required. Make a note of all relevant details.
9. Make a commitment to quality in everything you do. Do not make excuses for poor performance.
10. Remember that *poor outcome* (due to inherent risks and unpredictability of biological processes) is not the same as *poor performance*. Ensure that your patients and their families understand this well before any risky procedure is undertaken. You can guarantee performance but not the outcome.

HOW TO BUILD PATIENT TRUST ON THE FIRST VISIT

We all know that patient compliance is important to successful medical care. Physicians on average believe that about two-thirds of their patients are fully compliant. This is an overestimate. In some surveys, less than half the patients surveyed were compliant.

Patient compliance starts not after the patient returns home, but at the very first contact, s/he has with your office. How this first interaction develops very often decides how much your patients will comply with your treatment plans. Therefore, it is in the best interests of you and your patients' to realise the important role other staff can play in developing compliance. To enhance the quality of every patient visit, especially new patient visits, nothing should be left to chance. The first meeting needs to be planned carefully by physicians and their staff using the following points as a guide.

Appointment

New patients should, if possible, be scheduled for the lightest times of the day, and asked to come in 10 minutes before their appointment time. I call my new cases at 8.30 am, i.e. 45 minutes before a patient-crowd collects.

Welcome

The patient should be greeted warmly by the receptionist or other designated staff, who should introduce themselves first.

Information

After the introductions, the staff should explain any official procedures for this and future visits, such as the importance of bringing old healthcare records or a list of medications.

Collecting Patient Data

New patients need to know from the very beginning that you and your staff respect the confidential nature of their relationship with you. Personal information should never be taken orally in a crowded reception room, especially in specialities like psychiatry, andrology, gynaecology, venereology, etc.

Conducting the Patient for the Consultation

Many doctors may like to greet new patients in the privacy of examination room. This is an ideal time to develop rapport and further solidify a clinical relationship with the patient.

Meeting the Doctor

In routine cases, especially chronic diseases, the first visit with the doctor should be more of an introductory meeting to establish initial rapport. When an urgent problem has brought the patient, the doctor should deal with the immediate problem and ask the patient to book another appointment, when medical history and past treatments can be discussed in more detail. Broader the speciality, more important is this step.

Saying Goodbye

This step involves the patient, the doctor and the staff. When the medical component of the visit is over, you want them to leave with good feeling about your practice and to feel confident that they have found a competent physician who runs an efficient clinic. Walking with them to the door and opening it for them while saying goodbye to the patient and his/her attendants is an excellent gesture.

TEN TIPS TO RAPPORT BUILDING

Here are specific, common sense approaches, backed by research, to build a relationship with anyone:

Treat People Differently to Get Along Well

Among psychologists, the accepted major personality variables are the "Big 5":

- Extroversion-introversion
- Neuroticism
- Openness to experience
- Agreeableness
- Conscientiousness

These personality traits are far more comprehensive and psychologically valid than other personality systems like type A and B. Whatever may be the personality classification system you use, the point is to adjust your behaviour to match your patient's style. For example, a type A person, who talks fast, gets impatient if you do not get to the point soon enough. Type B, who prefers a slower pace, may get nervous if you are a Type A. If you match your patient's style, the first meeting will be smoother and is more likely to lead to a good rapport.

This advice to be a chameleon in terms of matching other people's styles could be questioned ethically. It is largely a matter of intentions. If behavioural matching (mirroring) is done to manipulate patients, it is part of charlatanism; if done just to build a better rapport and to make patients more comfortable, then it is a part of patient-centred practice (see Neuro-linguistic programming).

Reinforce Relationship

Patients reason that the more you invest in the relationship with them, the less likely you are to abandon them when they need you. New patients figure that if you are not persistent when you want them to enlist your services, you may not be around when you have them in your list.

Look for Reciprocity—Within Limits

Relationships are built from a two-way flow of reinforcement. The rhythm of responsiveness between two parties is as important in relationship building as in a conversation. If you do not respond to friendly overtures, you will break the rhythm.

In practice, this can be simple. If your conversations start as strictly clinical, add a more personal comment; your patients will respond if they are in tune with you. As a health professional, one should avidly develop *clinical* and *therapeutic* relationship with patients. One should be cautious in developing a *personal* relationship. One must avoid *intimate* relationship with patients. It is unethical unless you break the unequal professional-client relationship first. If any accusations are made later, you, as the dominant person in the dyad, shall be culpable even if the patient is a consenting adult.

Find Similarities in Personal or Professional Areas

This is a good common sense advice, supported by hundred of studies by psychologists such as Donn Byrne. While different people can get along well because they complement each other, research is overwhelming that similarity leads to liking. *In human relationships, "Like poles attract."*

Patients feel safer if you have things in common with them. Especially if you share values, they can understand you better and predict your decisions. If you share friends, you are less likely to exploit them because the word will spread to others.

Create Chances for Repeated Interaction

In general, people tend to like the persons they see the most. In other words, the more your patients get to see you, the more they would like it, unless you are reinforcing them negatively.

My experience is that with every new patient, it takes about three consultations to achieve a good rapport and a workable therapeutic relationship. People who do not like to see me—for whatever reasons—drop out after one or two consultations and the relationship never goes beyond a *clinical* (adult to adult) level.

Make Yourself "Attractive"

Unfair as it may be, physically attractive people tend to be liked more. Research has shown that good looks provide benefits in many contexts. Physically attractive doctors are perceived to be more intelligent, competent and successful. Again, attractive appearance has to be within ethical norms. Most patients expect only these: *an alert face and a clean white coat.* Flashy dress may be thought as a sign of frivolousness.

Give Items that Interests them

Most people appreciate the gesture, primarily because it shows that you are thinking about them and, secondly, because sometimes the material is of value. You may give free samples for trial, patient education brochures or even a toffee for very young patients.

Be Smarter in Handling Information

Use a reliable system to keep track of information. First, you have to collect information about your patients. Then, you have to recollect it. Fortunately, any of us can be a genius at remembering information by using a database. Even a paper and pencil system, reviewed before each consultation, can suffice.

For example, when a child with a pet named "Kitty", comes in for a consultation, the doctor's first question is not about her symptoms, but rather, "How is Kitty?" That one question personalises the interaction and puts her at ease. On the doctor's part, all it took was writing the cat's name on her chart during the previous visit. It could also be about a child's "best friend" or "best toy".

Show a Sense of Humour

Research shows that people like persons who have a sense of humour. Having a sense of humour does not mean you have to tell jokes; it means that *you are not grim about life*; you have a wry way of looking at the world and yourself. You use a little self-deprecating humour, especially if you have reached a high status. Your patients would feel better after being around you, not worse. So start spreading a little cheer from today.

Be Sincere, not a Phoney

Most books on how to make friends and influence people recommend doing things that do not match your real self. If you attract people by trying to be what you are not (a phoney), it may not lead to true rapport. It is up to you to reveal something about your true self to others, i.e. sincerity of purpose.

Closing Remarks

The tenth tip (*be sincere*) seems to be contrary to the first (*match your behaviour*) and sixth (*dress well*) tips. It is not so. Behaviour matching or being attractive reflects the art of communication for rapport building; being sincere refers to the professional and ethical commitment to an enduring doctor-patient relationship.

ADVANCED SKILLS

Dealing with Patient Personality Types

Not all patients are created equal. Their socio-economic, educational and personality development are vastly different. Once we accept them as our patients, they all deserve professional and courteous relationship with us, regardless of their idiosyncrasies. In doing so, we conform to the 'Justice and Equality' principle of professional ethics. Eight personality-types seen in patients and some tactics of dealing with them are discussed below:

Superior Type

Is arrogant and snobbish; feels invulnerable; often denies that the disease can cause any harm to him/her; feels important about self. A chief executive, a village chief, a head master and a god-man are some examples of persons who may present to you with a superior type of personality.

Tactics

- Readily acknowledge your patient's worth in his/her own field of expertise.
- Always maintain Adult-to-Adult type of conversation and transactions; avoid humour until you have a good rapport.
- Without sounding arrogant, strongly affirm your professional expertise, especially when challenged or accosted by the patient.
- Avoid 'Parent-Child' transactions (see Annexure - Transactional analysis).

Hysterical Type

Usually dramatises symptoms of illness but may even deny or repress facts related to diseases; flirtatious and seductive in behaviour; has underlying emotional insecurity and needs repeated reassurance. Boys and girls in their early teen may often appear to be of this type and may develop a 'crush' for their doctor. Other age groups may also present as dramatising type of patients.

Tactics

- Allow the patient to discuss his/her fears freely.
- Help distinguish facts from fantasies.
- Be generous in reassurance and emotional support.
- Discourage any emotional involvement.
- Guard against any unethical response to flirtatious or seductive appeal. The onus is on us, the professionals to do so in the unequal provider-client relationship.

Impulsive Type

Demands fast and easy solutions to health problems; has low threshold for frustration; often appears childish in outlook and rebellious or aggressive in health seeking behaviour.

Tactics

- Set firm limits—*do not permit undue expectations.*
- Hold the patient responsible for any impulsive action.
- Avoid open and direct confrontations as it may lead to unpleasantness and angry exchange of words.
- Avoid humour and jokes as the person may react violently to them.

Masochistic Type

Is long-suffering by own admission; sees the present illness as one more episode of life-long occurrences of unpleasant events. I see several harried housewives from the low-income group in this mould.

Tactics

- Do not avoid them it aggravates sickness and suffering.
- Do not adopt a nurturing parent role as it may worsen the illness-related masochism. Maintain an Adult-to-Adult type transaction.
- Avoid reinforcing the sick-role by showing undue sympathy. Use optimism and humour to cheer up the person.
- Set limits of health care responsibility or else they may end up becoming excessively dependent on you.
- Support and guide family members and caregivers at home who must deal with "poor me" masochism all the time. (See 'Existential position' in 'Transactional analysis').

Shy Type

Is reticent, seems to be aloof, silent and detached; underplays symptoms and illness; answers in a laconic way to open-ended questions. Female patients from conservative background commonly present this way.

Tactics

- Respect their need for privacy. (See 'Privacy' in chapter 1)
- Be friendly and empathetic but do not expect them to respond it is against their character to do so
- Play 'nurturing parent' role and see if your support works
- Asking questions (closed-ended probing questions) to derive more information
- Advice them to "Be prepared" for the next visit
- Encourage expressing "Concerns" (*vide infra* section III).

Suspicious Type

Is paranoid about being harmed, exploited or taken for a ride; tends to blame others for their illness and other problems in life.

Tactics

- Be friendly and open during the dyad.
- Maintain an Adult-to-Adult relationship in all transactions; any other role raises their suspicion.
- Avoid humour and cryptic comments.
- Inform all options fully.
- Acknowledge the need for circumspection and critical analysis in taking healthcare decisions. Encourage and coax them to clarify all their lingering doubts and objections; but be firm in your rebuttal and refutation basing them on solid evidence and undeniable facts (see 'Negotiating skills").

Controlling Type

Has an overriding need for control of all health problems by oneself; sees body parts and bodily functions as 'objects' to be under one's own control. Instead of saying, "I have headache", such a person may say, "My head gives me a lot of problems" or words to that effect.

Tactics

- Inform them methodically about the nature of illness and various management options.
- Include such patients in decision-making (see 'Informed decision-making' in chapter 6).
- Encourage patients and make them responsible for selfcare; they would appreciate that.
- Make them feel that they are in control of their illness or disability to the extent possible.
- Inform clearly the bodily functions and events that cannot be controlled by volition (the non-modifiable factors).

Dependent Type

Has an insatiable healthcare need; overly dependent on their doctors to solve all their problems, including non-medical ones; tax their doctors to the point of creating anger or frustration.

Tactics

- Show readiness and willingness to care for them.
- Interact in a direct and open way. Try to avoid Parent-Child transactions as it aggravates dependency.
- Set firm limits (time, availability, areas of healthcare under your responsibility, etc.)
- Avoid direct confrontation but turn responsibility for their behaviour back to them.
- Persuade them to be more autonomous and independent; appreciate and support their attempts to do so.

Uses and Limitations

Once you assign a patient to a type, your tactics for effectively dealing with them begin to form. However, you must be aware of the limitations of extrapolating these principles beyond a point. At times the initial impression may be wrong and mid-course corrections may have to be made. Some patients consulting you for a long time may evolve from one type to another, for example, a shy one to a dependent one.

Though, these principles help us to understand ourselves and others, common misuses include labelling patients and putting them into pigeonholes. We may then become numb to the richness of human interaction. In reality, there are more personality types in the world than there are people. (Remember that some of us have multiple personalities!)

Influence of Doctor's Personality

Doctors are also human beings with individual personality profiles. In a dyad, both personalities interact to create a variety of possible situations. It is beyond the scope of this book but left to the readers to imagine interesting combinations.

To sum up, People are wonderfully different. Enjoy the rich experience of each personality with which you interact.

FINE-TUNING YOUR LANGUAGE (NEUROLINGUISTIC PROGRAMMING)

You can learn to consciously control your communication skills by learning Neuro-Linguistic Programming (NLP). NLP explores how people create and maintain their thoughts and experiences (Steinbach, 1984). It has been described as "software for the brain." Information scientist Richard Bandler and linguistics professor John Grinder developed it in the early 1970's.

NLP is made up of the following elements:

- Physiology of communication (see chapter 1)
- Breathing (in tune with the other person)
- Conceptual quantity (see 'Conceptual Chunk' in chapter 5)
- Voice quality, tone and control (see 'Answering skills')
- Sensory language (see below).

Speaking a Patient's Language

This is psychologically sound as well as being considerate of what the patient can easily comprehend. For example, when talking with a production engineer, use engineering terms to explain diseases and treatment procedures, for example, "Your thyroid gland's *machinery has slowed down* and the *production* of thyroid hormone is grossly inadequate." The same message to a teacher may run thus: "Your thyroid has *failed*. It does not *obey the instructions* of its *master*, the pituitary gland."

When you use the language of your patient's profession—the acronyms, jargon, symbols and orientation—s/he will find it easy to absorb the information, to relate to you and to form a close rapport with you. You need a good general knowledge and creativity to master this art. Learn it by observing experienced clinicians.

In addition, most people have a preferred communication channel. It may be visual, auditory or action oriented. By keenly observing and listening to a patient, you can often find out a patient's favourite communication channel. By speaking the same language, you can develop a quick and easy rapport with the patient.

Visual Language

Observe your patient's eye movements. When talking with you, visually oriented patients will frequently look up, or allow their eyes to pan from left to right. Such eye movements mean that the patient is seeing with his or her mind's eye. This person uses his or her memory and imagination in a visual way. Other signs of visualisation include frequent blinking, closing the eyes and a glassy or unfocused look.

Listen for visual language. Patients who speak the visual language tend to use words like these frequently: *Look at; it appears; I see; observe; notice; from that angle; your viewpoint not clear, bright idea, etc.* Observe your patients' body language. They tend to dress better than others do in their socio-economic range.

Talking with Visually Oriented Patients

To successfully deal with a "visual-patient" requires using "visual words" in your talk, inviting the patient to use his or her mind's eye. For example:

- "Imagine how your abdomen will *look* like in a month from now."
- "Can you *see the expression* on your wife's face when you give her this good news that your tumour is benign and not a cancer?"
- "*Picture* the improved quality of life you would have after surgery and *see* if the benefits justify the risks."

Make liberal use of brochures, photographs, visual aids and computer screen or videotapes. They fix the patient's attention. Since you are using the patient's natural language, s/he gets a clear picture of your message.

Auditory Language

Observe your patients' eye movements; they provide the clues even with auditory people. The eye movements are not random movements. If you look closely at the patients while think and recall, they tend to look to their left and downwards; in addition, these patients tend to talk to themselves.

Observe their body language and voice. These patients touch their faces, tap their chins or rub their cheeks; they may be in the "telephone position" or sit like the famous 'thinker statue', which means they are talking to themselves, also known as *internal dialogue mode.* Studies show this applicable even in cultures where there are no telephones. The next time you rest your chin on your hands, check yourself by asking, "What am I telling myself?" If you make this a habit, you will develop a high degree of awareness of your internal dialogue.

Patients who are primarily sound-oriented tend to speak in an even and pleasant voice. You can occasionally hear them hum, whistle or make clicking sounds.

Listen for auditory language. Those preferring the auditory language tend to use words like these frequently: *Announce; ask for; sounds good; quietly; tell me; cry (for...); etc.*

Talking with Auditory People

Learn to speak the language of the sound-oriented patient. Do so by using the sound words. Some examples:

- "I am glad you are not *quiet* about your wife's illness but taking *sound* steps to cure the problem."
- "You should *hear* a good news from the laboratory regarding control of your blood sugar."

When called for, give your sound-oriented patient the chance to talk with a couple of satisfied patients who have similar problems. When s/he hears what these patients say, it will have a positive impact.

The Action and Feeling Language

Most of us like to watch others in action. We love to watch sports and action movies on TV. What is even more interesting to many are attractive TV commercials. By their very nature, all TV commercials use both visual and auditory channels. Study some good ones to find out what they do and how they do it: "*Reach out and touch...*" is action/feeling language, although it may only refer to a cell-phone. "*Go for it*" is pure action-feeling language and may refer to a shoe or a soft drink.

Action-feeling expressions abound in everyday language:

- "He is a pushy man."
- "They are on a fast track."
- "She is a go-getter."
- "Cloning and gene therapy—that is where the action is."

Some are old clichés; others are not. All have gusto and verve. They arouse people.

Observe your patient's eye movements. Action and feeling oriented patients frequently tend to look down and to the right, a characteristic that is associated with tuning into and sorting out one's feelings.

Listen for action-feeling language. Patients who are strongly action-feeling oriented use the following words frequently: *Active; affected; drives me; bearable; boils down to; run away; go away; fighting with; can handle, etc.*

Observe voice, breathing, body language and rate of speech. Action-feeling people tend to breathe fully and deeply, using a lot of gestures and body movement when speaking. They tend to speak somewhat slowly in low and resonant voices and frequently touch their clothing or their bodies. Patients who have a muscular body tend to be action-feeling persons. Later in life, they have a tendency to be overweight. Those people also reveal themselves by references to their hobbies (outdoor sports, travel, etc.) during medical interview.

Talking with Action-feeling Persons

To deal successfully with the action-feeling patient, use words that refer to movement, action and feeling. Let the patient get a feel for your service and realise how the planned procedure will work to his/her benefit.

An example: "The coronary bypass is aimed at *putting you back on your feet.*"

Involve your action-feeling patients physically whenever possible. Have them walk through the hospital or wards with you. When it is not possible to put the patient through an actual experience, you have a choice among various desktop demonstrations or talking about how other patients feel about using your service.

ELICITING UNVOICED CONCERNS

The importance of patients' involvement in decision-making is now accepted by the medical profession. For patients to be involved, their priorities must be identified and addressed. Most patients prefer doctors who discuss with them about all their (patients') problems but the patients are often passive and expect the doctor to initiate relevant query. Unequal power structure with the health professional holding the upper hand over the patient is the main reason for this. The onus is on the professional to take the initiative to elicit these concerns.

Moreover, many patients are reluctant to talk to family physicians about certain health issues that affect quality of life. A study by Street, et al. examined the factors that influence a patient's willingness to discuss about his/her overall well being, physical health, and psychosocial health. Patients were more willing to discuss all aspects.

i. When they believed that it was the doctor's job to ask about these issues and
ii. When they had a longer relationship with the doctor.

Agenda and Expectation

The concept of *patients' total agendas* is preferable to the concept of *patients' expectations. Agenda* includes all the reasons for clinical dyad and encompasses patients' ideas, concerns, and expectations. *Expectations* include those related to the clinical management as well as aspects concerning relationship with the doctor.

Levenstein, et al. introduced the concept of *agendas* as the key to understanding patients. They found that doctors failed to elicit patients' reasons for consulting and the cause of their worries in half the dyads. Campion, et al. showed that social and emotional agendas are underrepresented in the consultation. Doctors may overestimate the extent to which patients are primarily concerned with medical treatment rather than with gaining information and support. In any geriatric clinic, you will find a number of "elderly well" who visit regularly just for support and reassurance.

Voices of Medicine and Lifeworld

Study of *voiced* and *unvoiced* agendas reveals how patients communicate in consultations. During medical consultations, patients seem to have a limited autonomy to make requests but not to suggest solutions. However, outside medical consultations, these patients communicate well, revealing their feelings and their own ideas on their health problems, and voice opinions and possible criticisms of medical treatments. Mishler described these as two voices: *the voice of medicine,* in which the consultation is conducted, and *the voice of the Lifeworld,* which is largely left outside the consultation.

- The *voice of medicine* is characterised by medical terminology, objective descriptions of physical symptoms, and the classification of these within a reductionist biomedical model. The patient is commonly construed as a purely "biomedical" entity that is, a person with disconnected bodily symptoms, wanting a label for what is wrong and a prescription to put it right. Consequently, patients may feel that their voice is overridden, silenced, or stripped of personal meaning and social context.
- The *voice of patient's lifeworld,* on the other hand, is characterised by non-technical description of the subjective experience of illness within the context of the patient's everyday world.

Even within the framework of biomedical model, the patients do not often voice the following:

- Additional symptoms
- Previous treatment or self treatment
- Socio-economic context of illness, request for diagnosis
- Theories about diagnosis and worries about diagnosis or prognosis
- Prescription request or not wanting a prescription
- Reporting or discussing side effects.

While these items may be discussed in social dyads, they may remain unvoiced in medical dyads. In short, *patients behave as they believe patients are expected to "play the role" rather than as they would like to behave.* The onus seems to be on doctors to elicit patients' ideas and expectations thereby showing that the patients' co-provider role is a valuable and necessary contribution to the consultation. To achieve this, the doctors need to listen and ask the right questions. Some are listed below:

Eight Questions to Unravel "Patient Agenda"

(Those of the traditional medical history are not listed here)

- What made you decide to fix this appointment? Why have you come to consult me now?
- What do you think is wrong with you? (*Probe for fears about illness*)
- Do you have any ideas about the best way to treat your symptoms or illness? (*Prompt: is there any type of treatment or medicine you do not want?*)
- What did you do about your symptoms or illness before you made this appointment to see the doctor? (*Probe: did they talk it over with anyone, ask anyone for advice, or take anything for it?*)
- What do you hope I/we can do for you?
- Is there anything you do not want the doctor to do for you? (*Probe for any type of treatment or medicine not wanted*)
- Often people are expecting one of the following when they visit the doctor. Are you expecting any of these? If so, which ones? (Show card, which lists reassurance, advice, information, diagnosis, finding out what is wrong, referral to a specialist, tests, investigations, medical certificate, sick note, medical check up, a prescription for tablets or medicines, a repeat prescription for tablets or medicine)
- Do you wish to talk about any other problems?

Doctors who adopt a *paternalistic approach* may have little interest in discussing patient concerns expressed "in the voice of the life-world." Those who adopt the *informed approach* permit the patients a more active role in defining the health problem and in deciding the appropriate management. Only those who follow the *shared approach* commit themselves to an interactive relationship with their patients in developing a plan that is consistent with patients' values and preferences for management of the illness.

To sum up, if the doctors' dyadic behaviour changes, then the patients can also be facilitated to change. While paying attention to the unique experience of illness of each patient (*life-world*), we should not lose our focus on the disease (*medical world*). We have to learn to take the patient along the path of scientific medicine with his/her full co-operation. This would be possible if we cultivate the fine art of unravelling the patient's agenda.

SUMMARY

Learn to speak the patients' language. Two ways of doing so are: i) to use words and jargon related to your patients' job and hobby and ii) to detect and use the preferred information channel of your patients (visual, auditory or action-feeling). These sound natural and intuitively make sense to them. This would lead to a better doctor-patient relationship. Integrity and technical skill are the main qualities that differentiate between a sound and a mediocre professional, form the foundation of lasting provider-client relationships. Do what you say you will do. Establish a proven record of accomplishment of honouring your commitments. People will take notice. They will respect you, believe you and develop faith in all that you do. In turn, you will believe more in yourself and in your abilities.

BIBLIOGRAPHY

1. Barry CA, Bradley CP, Britten N, Stevenson FA, Barber N. Patients' unvoiced agendas in general practice consultations. *BMJ* 2000;320:1246-50.
2. Cathy Charles, Amiram Gafni, Tim Whelan Editorial: How to improve communication between doctors and patients. *BMJ* 2000;320:1220-21.
3. Integrity and client centeredness Sales Doctors Communication series (1996)- Bruce R Wares.
4. Nicky Britten, Fiona A Stevenson, Christine A Barry, Nick Barber, Colin P Bradley. Misunderstandings in prescribing decisions in general practice: qualitative study. BMJ. 2000;320:484-8.
5. Rick Crandall. Secrets to Building Relationships. www.salesdoctor.com.
6. Steinbach AM. Neurolinguistic Programming: A Systematic Approach to Change. Can Fam Physician 1984;30:147-150 available at http://www.ncbi.nlm.nih.gov/pmc/articles/PMC2153995/pdf/canfamphys00215-0149.pdf *(accessed on 18-09-2010).*
7. Street RL Jr, Cauthen D, Buchwald E, Wiprud R. Patients' predispositions to discuss health issues affecting quality of life. Family Medicine 1995;27:663-70.
8. Thom DH. Campbell B. Patient physician trust: An exploratory study. Journal of Family Practice 1997;44:169-76.

SECTION 1

PRACTICAL EXERCISES

1. *Perception of Patient's Personality* (*Simulation Role-play*)
   Different personality types can be enacted or shown on video. The students learn how to interact with each type of personality.
2. *Using Sensory Channel* (*Group Discussion with Video triggers*)
   From several dyads in TV serials or films, short video triggers can be selectively edited to reveal the fine art of Neuro-linguistic programming. Many talented directors and scriptwriters build these into the dyads. A batch of students can observe, discuss and learn various ways of communicating by visual, auditory or action-feeling language.
3. *Rapport Building skills* (*Simulation Role-play*)
   Students pair off. Clinical situations are assigned to each pair. These should relate to common occurrences in clinical practice. The 'doctor' talks with the 'patient' who keeps track of the doctor's behaviour and the mode of conveying information. (A third student may play the role of 'observer' to note the details of the dyad).

   In the plenary session, the tutor can discuss the observations of all the groups and suggest ways to improve rapport-building skills. If video recording is available, feedback session can be more objectively discussed.
4. *Eliciting 'Unvoiced concerns' or Patient-agenda* (*Simulation Role-play*)
   Use simulated patients with hidden agenda. An example is a newly married man with 'performance anxiety' presenting with sympathotonic symptoms like palpitation, tremors, etc. Students have to ask the '8-questions' and unravel the unvoiced concern.

CHAPTER

8

Counseling Skills

The ultimate humanistic goal of counseling is to help people recognize and accept their own internal worth and to integrate their self-image and their learned behaviours (knowledge, attitude & actions) to truly reflect their goodness as beautiful, loving people.

—D Santoro

COUNSELING THEORY

What is Counseling in Healthcare?

Counseling is a process of initiating change towards healthy living or healing, in which people (individuals, groups, couples, and families) are helped to:

- Express themselves (catharsis) in a safe, supportive, collaborative, non-judgmental climate;
- Identify, sort-out, clarify their problems and deepen awareness of past & present;
- Identify maladaptive and non-helpful coping patterns;
- Adopt, where appropriate, more helpful coping skills;
- Identify and achieve goals that are important to them.

Simply stated, counseling is any relationship in which one person is helping another person to better understand and solve some problem. Teachers, friends and relatives, priests and many others provide a type of counseling. Counselors have a broad range of experience in developing "helping relationships" and working with many different situations. In counseling, a *counselor* helps the *counseled* look for what s/he finds 'good' in her/himself. The good can then be used as a basis for things s/he would like to change.

Counseling Approaches: Formal

Cognitive Approach

This is based on the principle that *our thoughts are directly connected to how we feel.* Therapists in the cognitive field, work with clients to solve present day problems by helping them to identify distorted thinking that causes emotional discomfort.

The focus is on, *"What's wrong with my present thinking that it causes me distress."* There's little emphasis on the historical root of a problem. Cognitive approaches include a collaborative relationship between client and therapist, and are best known for treating mild depression, anxiety, and anger problems.

Gestalt Therapy

"Gestalt," a German word meaning "whole," operates as a therapy by guiding the person to gain insight. Therapists help clients to be attentive to all parts of themselves: posture, breathing, methods of movement, etc. An emphasis is placed on personal responsibility for one's own well being. The focus is on, "*Why it happens?*"

Behavioral Therapy

This is based on the premise that primary learning comes from experience. The initial concern is to help the patient analyze behavior, define problems, and select goals. The focus is on "*What to do?*" rather than why it happens. Therapy often includes homework, behavioral experiments, role-playing, assertiveness training, and self-management training. Like its cognitive therapy, it utilizes collaboration between client and therapist, is usually of short duration and helps in effecting behavioral changes.

Psychoanalytic Therapy

The so-called "talking therapy" involves analyzing the root causes of behavior and feelings by exploring the unconscious mind and the conscious mind's relation to it. Many variations have evolved since Freudian days, e.g., Hypnotherapy, object-relations, Jungian etc. One thing they all have in common is that they deal with unconscious motivation. Usually the duration of therapy is lengthy; however, many modern therapists adopt psychoanalytic techniques for short-term counseling.

Counseling Approaches: Non-Formal

The methods discussed above need formal training. The following approaches are instinctive and can be adopted by clinicians to counsel their patients.

Adlerian

Considered the first "*common sense*" therapy, its basic premise is that human beings are always "becoming," that we're always moving towards the future, and our concerns are geared towards our subjective goals rather than an objective past. We are constantly aiming towards what Adler calls *superiority*. When we have unrealistic or unattainable goals, this can lead to self-defeating behaviors and discouragement, which may foster neurosis, psychosis, substance abuse, criminal behavior, or suicide. *The focus is on self-realization, acceptance and adaptation.* The role of the counselor is to help the client

- Identify mistaken goals,
- Do away with self-centredness, egotism, and isolation, and
- To develop positive, meaningful interpersonal relationships.

Medical professionals can adopt this 'common sense model' to counsel patients with self destructive behavior like ingesting poison, deliberate non-compliance, etc.

Person-Centred (Rogerian)

Founded by Carl Rogers in the 1940's, like Adlerian therapy, a basic premise is that we are all "becoming;" we are all moving towards self-actualization. He believed that each of us has the innate ability to reach our full potential. As infants, we are born with it, but because of early experiences, we may lose our connection to it. The self-concept we develop in response to our early experiences may tend to alienate us from our true self.

In this theory, there is no such thing as mental illness. It is just a matter of being disconnected from our self-potential. This therapy is often considered the most optimistic approach to human potential.

This model is based on a nurturing counselor-client relationship. The counselor provides the conditions necessary for the client's growth—genuineness, unconditional positive regard, and empathic understanding. If the process works, the client moves back towards self-actualization. *The focus is on nurturing the patient to adopt positive self-image and practice useful coping strategies.*

Solution-Focused Brief Therapy

This short-term counseling is based on:

- Focusing on solutions instead of problems
- Exceptions suggest solutions, i.e. To a patient who says, "I am always afraid of getting a heart attack," ask, "Think of a time when you were not afraid of it." Based on that, devise possible solutions
- Change is occurring all the time and small changes lead to large changes
- People have all they need to solve their problems.

The premise is that if one follows these assumptions in a step-wise manner, s/he can find quick solutions to whatever they might be facing.

Solution focussed counseling quite useful in helping patients with chronic stress related problems like tension headache, migraine, irritable bowel syndrome etc., to help them to get on with their lives accepting their symptoms and coping with them effectively. Initially, three consultations are required to make some impact and then periodic review session keep the patient on the right track.

Client's Responsibilities in Counseling

Clients' main responsibilities in counseling are to talk about what is bothering them as openly and honestly as they can, and complete any tasks or "homework" assignments they may be asked to do. Most counseling will require them to try something new or a "different approach." Another thing the counselor will expect, is for them to have an open mind and try things without jumping to conclusions. They are also expected to let their counselor know if their problems are being solved or not.

Common Difficulties in Counseling

One of the most difficult steps in counseling is to help the patient realise that s/he needs counseling. Once this decision has been made, the mechanics for change have been set in motion. The process of changing the way your patient think, feel, or behave, one usually must coax them to try out new ways of doing things. This can make both parties anxious or frustrated. Moreover, defense mechanisms of the patient often surface and interfere with progress.

Defense Mechanisms

One uses their defenses to distance themselves from distressing feelings and maintain emotional stability. Our defense patterns began in childhood when they prevented us from becoming overwhelmed with anxiety. As adults, we outgrow the need for such a defense but they may persist. Defenses are not conscious excuses to avoid problems. They are usually subconscious. Part of counseling is to help the patients identify their defense. If they can discover it, they can replace maladaptive ones with healthier ones.

Some commonly used unhelpful defenses are:

Rationalization

Providing explanatory excuses justifying inconsistent or irrational behavior, without being aware of it, e.g., an alcoholic saying, "I take it only to induce a good sleep."

Minimizing

Protecting oneself from worry or anxiety by viewing significant problems as being less important than they actually are, e.g. an alcoholic saying, "It is within safe limits."

Externalization

Belief in outside forces or circumstances as the cause of one's self-destructive behaviors. This defense mechanism allows one to avoid accepting responsibility, e.g., an alcoholic saying, "My horrible job is the reason for my habit. It helps me survive one more day at the workplace."

Projection

This is similar to externalization, but here, the attribution of one's own undesirable traits or thoughts is onto another person, e.g., an alcoholic blaming his wife for his habit.

Intellectualization

Using *deflecting behavior* (a lengthy argument or small details) to distract from the task at hand, e.g., an academician, who is an alcoholic, lecturing about various 'good' effects of alcohol on lipid metabolism, etc.

Displacement

Redirecting negative emotions like anger from its source onto other persons, objects, or ideas, e.g., an incompetent man redirecting his negative emotions by beating his wife and children.

Undoing

Engaging in behavior intended to make amends for previously unacceptable thoughts, feelings, or actions, e.g., a housewife, who has contemplated suicide, realizing her folly, cooks a special dinner for the family.

Note: This is not to be confused with actual and direct amends made to persons one may have harmed.

Fantasy

Escaping from an unpleasant situation by daydreaming, or not paying attention.

Acting-out

Impulsive acting without reflection or apparent regard for negative consequences, e.g., a newly married wife consuming poison because her husband left her at home and went to a movie with his friends (by the way, a true story).

Regression

Returning to a less mature level of behavior, e.g., a teenage boy, when faced with a crisis, acting like a 5-year old.

Passive Aggression

Indirectly and unassertively expressing aggression towards others. This is quite common in India where repression is culturally well accepted. Non-compliance is the most common form seen in our patients.

An understanding of the various types of unhelpful and maladaptive defense mechanisms may help to counsel the patients better.

COUNSELING—PRACTICE

> *Words of comfort, skillfully administered are the oldest therapy known to man.*
> - Louis Nizer.

Clinical counseling is a process of helping the patients (by interview techniques) to make sound and rational decisions based on an examination of relevant facts and deriving possible options. Examples of counseling in family planning (to understand the procedural elements), genetic counseling (to understand the underlying principles), nutritional counseling (to recognize various styles) and behavior change counseling are discussed below:

Family Planning (FP) Counseling

Family Planning (FP) Counseling aims to help clients to make voluntary, informed and well-considered decisions about their fertility and contraceptive options. The counseled clients should be able to:

- Decide whether to practice or not to practice FP
- Choose a FP method that is convenient and suitable to their needs and situation
- Practice the chosen FP method safely and effectively.

General Principles

i. Every client is unique. Therefore, the counseling approach should be individualized.

ii. The client has the right to make an informed and voluntary choice about whether to use a family planning method and if so, what method to use.
iii. The counselor should be objective and a non-judgmental in dealing with a client.
iv. The counselor should respect the confidentiality of a client.

Element of Counseling: The "GATHER Approach"

i. Greet clients
- Friendly welcome
- Treat client with respect
- Arrange for privacy

ii. Ask clients about their family planning needs
- The client's medical history
- Previous FP experience
- FP knowledge
- Concerns about FP
- Desire to use/switch FP methods
- Preferred method

iii. Tell clients about relevant family planning methods
- Information about availability of family planning services
- Referral services
- Other relevant information

iv. Help clients decide which method they want
- Listening skills of the counselor
- Tone of voice and choice of words (see note on "mitigated directives")
- Discussion about the client's health condition
- Probing into the client's reasons for seeking family planning
- Discussion on partner's attitude
- Clarifications on the client's concerns
- Explanation about the results of tests or physical examinations
- Encouraging the client to participate in the decision-making

v. Explain how to use the chosen method
- Explanation given about the methods
- Use of information materials
- Efforts to correct misconceptions
- Overall attitude towards the client
- Assurance given to return for any problems related to method choice/use

vi. Return visit (plan)
- Arrangement made for return visit
- Referral for FP or other health services.

Mitigated directives: These are suggestions such as, "Maybe you could try these", as opposed to such assertive directives as, "Try these." It has been argued that women offer more mitigated directives and more general markers of tentativeness and that this results in greater compliance. Both men and women professionals should learn to use mitigated directives.

Genetic Counseling

Use a Non-directive Approach

Consanguineous marriages are common in India and many of them are at genetic risk for diseases. Since they are already married, directive or judgmental type of counseling will only make them feel guilty or stupid. They will simply stop consulting the counselor. Non-directive counseling is appropriate in dealing with them.

Anticipate Logical Mismatch

While discussing risks of genetic diseases and ways of prevention, expect a mismatch between *medical logic* (defective baby is a medical failure and a folly) and *lay logic* based on hope, religious beliefs etc. Elicit their values and beliefs and be ready to clarify and counsel.

Take the Clients Seriously

Just because of any such logical mismatch that may make the couple's decision 'foolish' from medical view point do not make flippant remarks; take them seriously.

Respect Couple's Informed Decision

Respect the couple's informed decision, even if goes against medical logic. An example: A 35-year-old primigravida is counseled on the risk of baby having Down's syndrome and ways of detecting it by amniocentesis. She says, "I do not want to harm my baby by invasive procedures. If the baby is normal and amniocentesis initiates abortion, I can never forgive myself. God has finally answered my prayers and made this happen. He will decide if my baby will be normal or otherwise."

In this instance, lay logic is willing to face the risk based on faith in God. Medicalizing such situations is perhaps unwise. Striking a partnership deal is a way out.

Strike a Partnership Deal

If your rapport with the couple is good, strike a partnership deal by saying, "You are the experts on your unborn baby; I have expertise in genetic diseases. But our goal is same: your baby should be well. So why don't we pool our resources together and do our best for the baby instead of confronting with mismatched logic?"

Use Shared Model of Decision Making

Try to adopt a shared decision making based on consensus. Some couples may want autonomy in the final decision; then use informed decision-making model. By creative problem solving, try to accommodate couples' wishes within a rational medical framework.

An example: To a couple, who do not want invasive diagnostic procedures done on the foetus, you may ask, "If I can use a safe non-invasive method like ultrasound scanning, will you accept it? I do want to make sure your baby does not have any major defect incompatible with life. Then all your prayers and the long wait for 40 weeks will amount to nothing. Why not make sure that your baby is at least grossly normal?"

Nutritional Counseling Styles

In a Dutch study of general practitioners (GP), five styles of nutritional communication were identified, *viz.* informational, reference, motivational, confrontational and holistic style (van Dillen, 2006).

Some examples of different nutrition communication styles as explained by the counseling GP:

i. *Informational style*: "I tell the patient that he should eat less fat, but I leave it to him." Or "I have got a lot of education materials to give them to study at home."
ii. *Reference style*: "Several times you have to say: go to the dietician and let her analyze." Or "If there is a problem with weight or sugar, then I call the dietician."
iii. *Motivational style*: "I try hard to convince them, if they are willing to listen, that they can extend their life by 10 more years and see if they are really motivated."
iv. *Confrontational style*: "I check their weight and height and then I show them a BMI table which shows that they are in a high risk area." Or "I warned them several times about coronary risk, but some obese patients turn out to be stubborn."
v. *Holistic style*: "At first visit I discuss BMI and I show them that they are at risk. I ask them to keep up a diary of diet, exercise and body weight, so that we get a better view of their lifestyle."

Behavior Change Counseling by Motivational Interviewing

Motivational interviewing (MI) is a directive, client-centered counseling style for promoting behavior change by helping clients to explore and resolve their ambivalence to accepting lifestyle modifications. Behavior change counseling, derived from motivational interviewing, is a patient-centered, directive therapy used to address high risk behaviors (Emmons & Rollnick, 2001).

Inappropriate assumptions on behavior change are common and include the following:

- This person *wants* to change
- This patient's health is the prime motivating factor for him/her
- Patients are either motivated to change, or not (all or none)
- If he or she does not decide to change, the consultation has failed
- A tough approach is always best
- I am the expert and he/she must follow my advice for his/her own wellness.

An effective behavior change counselor must eschew such assumptions.

The Spirit of Motivational Interviewing

Motivation to change should be elicited from the client, not imposed by the counselor. The counselor gives directives to help the client examine and resolve ambivalence. It is the client's task, not the counselor's, to articulate and resolve his/her ambivalence. Direct persuasion, in which rational arguments for change are presented to the client by the expert, is not an effective method for resolving ambivalence.

Components of a Motivational Interview

i. Establish rapport to understand patient's concerns and circumstances.
ii. Raise the topic, say smoking as a high-risk behavior, and get patient acceptance to talk about the topic.

iii. Make the patient aware of consequences of the behavior, and share your concerns as a healthcare provider.
iv. Assess readiness to change behavior and offer advice accordingly:
   - Not ready to change: "What would it take to get you to consider thinking about a change?"
   - Unsure: "What are the things you don't like about this (issue/topic)? And what are the things that you like about it."
   - Ready: "Here are some options for change. What do you think would work best for you?."
v. Assure the patient that ongoing support is available.

SUMMARY

Good counseling skills are cultivated over years of practice. Regardless of the medical specialty of a doctor, the ability to counsel effectively is an asset that would contribute to a win-win partnership between the doctor and the patient.

BIBLIOGRAPHY

1. Emmons KM, and Rollnick S. Motivational Interviewing in Health Care Settings: Opportunities and Limitations. Am J Prev Med. 2001;20:68-74.
2. Atkin K, et al. Screening and counselling for Sickle cell Disorder and Thalassaemia. Soc Sci Med. 1998;47:1639-51.
3. van Dillen SME, Hiddink GJ, Koelen MA, de Graaf C, van Woerkum CMJ. Identification of nutrition communication styles and strategies: A qualitative study among Dutch GPs. Patient Education and Counseling. 2006;63:74–83.
4. Various articles on counseling in http://www.allaboutcounseling.com/ (accessed on 18-09-2010).

PRACTICAL EXERCISES

Role-plays

Demonstration

Experienced clinicians will demonstrate counseling skills in simulated situations. Common themes like smoker with chronic bronchitis, obesity with impaired glucose tolerance, lifestyle modifications in a patient with hypertension, migraine, asthma or epilepsy, genito-urinary hygiene for a patient with recurrent urinary infection etc. For variety, each of the counseled (simulated patient) can adopt a different defense position.

Practice

Students pair off, adopt various roles of counselor and counseled and practise counseling skills under observation and guidance by tutors. It is preferable to adopt micro-training strategy: feedback is given on the procedural steps (as in GATHER approach for family-planning counselling), on the principles and tactics used as in Genetic counseling, diet advice using different counseling styles and on the effectiveness of motivational interview technique for behavior change. The relevant parts of the text can be converted to a checklist or a 3 point rating scale.

CHAPTER

9

Skills of Persuasion

Patience and perseverance have a magical effect before which difficulties disappear and obstacles vanish.

—John Quincy Adams

Most young doctors assume that patients will avidly follow medical advice because they want to get better. In reality, patient's acceptance of medical advice is not that simple or straightforward. We need all our skills of persuasion to coax them to accept what they really need. Persuasion is an art and a skill that can be cultivated.

THE ART OF PERSUASION

How do you make your therapeutic advice persuasive? Will appeals to reason alone make your patients to comply with your advice and adhere to it? Do you need to stir their emotions, too? How important are other intangible factors, like your credibility and perceived integrity? Is there a "formula" for crafting a persuasive talk?

These questions—critical to anyone who has to advise others - have deep historical roots. Aristotle (4th century BC) discussed the puzzle of persuasion in his classic treatise, *The Rhetoric*. In that work, he sought to discover the elements of persuasion by distilling this abstract and amorphous subject into its fundamental components. He said that persuasion comprised of three essential elements: *Ethos* (ethics or character), *Logos* (logic), and *Pathos* (passion or emotion); in order to be persuasive, a speaker must embody character, logic and passion. All three elements are necessary; none can do the job alone.

Ethos

Ethos is the cornerstone of persuasion. Aristotle suggested a simple test: Does the speaker personify good character, good judgement, and good will? If you want to persuade a patient, you must first establish yourself as a professional of integrity and ethics.

For the health professional, however, establishing ethos means more than just showing personal integrity; it is also essential to convey relevant clinical skills and experience, outstanding knowledge of the subject, and solid consultative judgement. Patients are looking for more than honesty—they want expert problem-solvers.

Ethos is an elusive quality, but it can be developed and strengthened. Trial lawyers prepare witnesses to speak with sincerity and conviction, and you can use their methods. Practice your therapeutic advice while your peers observe (or record it on a videotape) and then ask your colleagues to criticise you. Do you come across as a credible, conscientious problem-solver? Or do you seem more like an advertiser? Refine your style until you convey honesty, integrity, and experience. Where there is no trust, there is no rapport or compliance.

For example, if you are a smoker and your patient is aware of it, your efforts at persuading him to give up smoking may not succeed because of the "preach-practice paradox."

Logos

It is apparent that logos is a central component of persuasion. Too many professionals presume that logic is its only component. A lengthy detailed advice, no matter how well-structured, is unconvincing. It is perhaps a paradox, but an effective advice must be more than simply logical—it must appeal to common sense. To do this, your advice should be:

- Clear, simple, and direct
- Systematic and easy to follow
- Expressed in the patient's own terms
- Tailored to the patient's real needs
- Supported by solid and memorable examples
- Easy to visualize (illustrated, where possible)
- As brief as possible

Make your central argument clear, concrete, and concise. Relating a relevant anecdote is a good way to hit these targets. Patients, like other humans, are narrative-oriented. A brief, story told in simple, concrete terms appeals to their sense of logic, while abstract, complex pitches do not. Always try to craft your advice to match the logical sophistication of your patients. Keep it organized and systematic, but keep it simple. (see 'conceptual chunk')

For example, in trying to persuade a patient to give up smoking, one has to use simple but effective narratives that may act as motivators or revelations. Conversational tone should be one of the 'adult to adult sharing of views' rather than that of 'parental preaching to a rebellious child'.

Pathos

While advising, health professionals commonly forget that patients are humans too. If patients were like robots, logic and statistics would be sufficient to do the job; but patients are human beings. No matter how sophisticated and hard-nosed they try to be, they are not motivated by logic alone. The notion that emotions and logic are separate forces that function independently in opposite cerebral hemispheres is well-accepted and reassuring but untrue in real world. In the patient's mind, reason and emotion overlap, with the pathos always shading logos.

Harnessing Pathos: How can you put pathos to work in your therapeutic advice to your patients?

Firstly, learn to speak with passion and conviction. Use strong images and examples to help your patients visualize your advice to solve their problem and making their life healthier, easier, or of better quality. Encourage them to "visualize" the results beforehand, and "experience" the rewards.

For example, when I talk to patients who need to give up smoking, I use a set of anecdotes based on my earlier cases; I choose the most relevant one in terms of age, smoke-related diseases and outlook, and narrate it with pathos. From the patient's body language, it is possible to know if you are getting through to them.

Secondly, go beyond the patient's actual health needs and consider broader, human issues. Try to uncover the patient's felt needs and goals. For example, when a clear cut case of migraine feels the need to get a CT scan done to rule out *brain cancer*, we have to explain why it is not in his/her interest to get it done. Otherwise, s/he may not be persuaded and may seek another opinion.

Until you convince a patient that his/her perceived needs are being taken care of in your follow up advice, persuasion may not succeed. Smokers commonly state that they need their daily puff for various reasons, like mental agility, to move their bowels or to keep their appetite down. If you convince them that you will devise safer methods to meet their felt needs, they may consider giving up smoking.

Thirdly, unearth the hidden emotional issues driving the patient and then use these strategically as tools of persuasion. Often, smoking against the wishes of the family members becomes a way of self-assertion; in such cases, more the family pressure, more is the resistance. The patient and the spouse are counseled about this hidden emotional issue. At times, they are suggested that if the spouse were to ask him to smoke more, he may actually rebel against it and stop smoking! If the patient is past 60 years, One may say, "Why don't you retire from this also? Do you want to be remembered by your grand children as '*cigarette grandpa*'?" A retired school teacher was moved to tears and stopped smoking from that day. In a given case, one can not be sure what tactic will work; one has to creatively keep trying several of them.

To sum up, when you try to persuade a patient, remember Aristotle's classic tools of persuasion: ethos, logos, and pathos. They still work! Be creative and exploit their persuasive potential fully.

PRACTICE OF PERSUASION

Learning the Techniques of Persuasion

- Know your audience and tailor your message accordingly
- Consider how to make yourself more persuasive, e.g. appearance
- Encourage audience participation
- Keep the message simple and straightforward
- Repetition is a useful technique
- Consider providing written handouts to back up a visual presentation
- Provide practical details so that the patient knows what to do
- The more thought and effort you put into the session, the more they will retain the message.

Too many health promotion efforts have disregarded basic techniques of persuasion and the lessons to be learned from advertising and psychology. Positive attribution may be more effective than persuasion in changing behavior.

Attribution Versus Persuasion

In terms of transactional analysis, persuasion reinforces "You are not OK; Why don't you try to be OK?" position. Positive attribution reinforces "You are OK. You can live up to it" position. Negative attribution reinforces "You are not OK. You are bound to fail unless you evolve" position. (See Annexure 1)

A study (Miller et al. 1975) compared the relative effectiveness of an attribution strategy with a persuasion strategy in changing behavior. An attribution group was repeatedly told that *they were neat and tidy* people. A persuasion group was repeatedly told that *they should be neat and tidy*, and a control group received no treatment. Attribution proved considerably more effective in modifying behavior. The study also revealed that attribution of ability was as effective as an attribution of motivation.

Persuasion often suffers because it involves a negative attribution (a person should be what he is not), while attribution generally gains because it disguises (a person should live up to his/her positive attributes) persuasive intent.

Use of Fear in Persuasion

Many health promotional messages are designed to persuade by eliciting fear, yet the use of fear is often ineffective in achieving the desired change in behavior. Fear that lacks direction and purpose may only challenge the audience to adopt risk-taking behavior. Such campaigns often fail and may even be counterproductive.

Fear is likely to be effective if you allow the desired behavior to be rewarded by a reduction in the level of fear. This entails five requirements:

- The adverse event upon which the fear is based should appear a likely threat, e.g. risk of HIV in unsafe sex
- Onset of fear should occur before the desired behavior is offered as a solution, e.g. the threat of HIV-AIDS in unsafe sex must induce fear in the audience before the solution of safe sex practices is offered.
- A specific desired behavior should be offered as part of the campaign, e.g. use of condoms
- The degree of fear elicited should be such that the desired behavior is perceived to substantially reduce the fear of perceived threat, e.g. spermicidal condom reducing HIV risk to negligible level
- Fear should not induce panic or shame. If the fear is overwhelming, stigmatization or fatalism may supervene and prevent any behavioral change. This has happened in many anti-HIV campaigns
- Reduction of fear (and threat perception) should occur as reinforcement for the desired behavior, confirming its effectiveness.

In general, a positive reinforcement approach may prove to be more effective than the use of fear.

The 'Sleeper Effect' (Why Persuasion may not Last)

The sleeper effect in persuasion is a delayed increase in the impact of a message that is accompanied by a discounting cue. When the message ('smoke tobacco') and discounting cue ('tobacco is harmful') have opposite and near-equal immediate impact, the message may seem to have been neutralized. Due to the differential decay of the two (the message and the cue), the stronger message regains its persuasive appeal. The sleeper effect occurs only if the impact of the discounting cue decays faster than that of the message. Then with passage of time, the main message ('the sleeper') regains more and more of its appeal.

Anti-smoking warnings have low impact due to 'sleeper effect' exploited by the advertisers. While pro-smoking imagery is very strong in its audio-visual appeal and impact, the discounting cue of statutory warning is displayed in an insignificant manner (color, font, no audio, etc). Therefore, in time, the statutory warnings fade away and only the promotional effect remains.

The sleeper effect may explain why many patients, who initially comply with your advice, go back to 'bad old ways.' While your advice fades away, the attraction for addictions may win over the patients. It is essential to reinforce persuasive messages repeatedly if they have to leave a lasting impact on the patients.

Persuading a Procrastinator

Most Indian patients are still dependent on their doctors for advice. So they do not openly disagree with the doctors' advice. Instead, they procrastinate and "sit on the fence" without taking healthcare decisions. This is a form of passive rejection. In our experience, "let me think it over" comes up more than any other excuse. There is a way to handle that objection. Rather than leaving it to the patients to sort out all the options for decision by themselves, provide them with a model that makes it easier to make up their mind.

Overcome "I'll have to think it over" by starting with this response: "Yes. All decisions should be made only after careful consideration. Let us discuss it now. There are three things which concern most people when they consider major healthcare decisions..."

Pull out a piece of paper and write:

1. Hospital
2. Service (Treatment procedure)
3. Cost of treatment

Leave some space under each item. After writing the three points, continue talking to the patient. If the patients do not like the hospital, they will not get admitted. It applies to the service also. If they do not like it, they will not get admitted. If the cost is not affordable, there is no way they can get treated there. Discuss these under each of the three headings. At the end, the sheet of paper will look like this:

1. Hospital:
   - Can they deliver care?
   - Are they reliable?
   - Will they be there to follow up and help?
   - (Additional items)
2. Service (Treatment procedure):
   - Will it help?
   - Will the results last?
   - Will it make a difference? (risk versus benefit)
   - (Additional items)
3. Cost of treatment:
   - Can I afford it?
   - Is it good value for the money? (cost versus benefit)
   - (Additional items)

At the end of this discussion, when a patient understands how well the hospital could satisfy his/her criteria for quality healthcare, proceed with the following three questions, pausing just long enough to get an agreement on each:

- Is this the sort of hospital (healthcare facility) where you would be happy to get treated?
- Is the quality of service and expertise acceptable to you?
- Regarding the expenses, the estimated cost of Rupees (x) includes ... (give a detailed list of all the items that are part of the service)
- Close the discussion by enquiring, "Have I cleared all your doubts?"
- When s/he says the final yes, continue with your advice for the next steps in the treatment procedure.

Remember that despite your best efforts, persuasion may not succeed because, in addition to your credibility and the strength of evidence of the disease, two other factors influence patient's perception and his/her acceptance of your suggestions.

Table 9.1: Interplay of factors that influence persuasion

	Subjective feeling (illness) ↓	
Doctor's credibility →		← Others' opinion and advice
	↑ Evidence and logic (disease)	

Coaxing a Strong Yes from Your Patient

Once you are aware of the variations in "yes", you should try and figure out the value of your patient's affirmative statements (see '4+ Yes' in chapter 5). If the value is not 3+ or more persuasion may not have succeeded. You should double check with the patient why they are not whole hearted in saying "yes" and clarify any misunderstanding or lingering doubts they may have. When I pick out a "1+ yes" in a patient and enquire if s/he is still not fully convinced, the patient is often stunned at how I could read their mind. It is not difficult if you train yourself to pick out the "Yes that does not mean yes."

Persuading for Organ Donation

In order to persuade possible donors to register for organ donation, you need to realize what motivates those who actually register their names. There are seven common motivating factors:

i. *Altruism*: The donor feels, "I feel fortunate to be able to help."
ii. *Normative motive*: "I have been brought up like that—to be of help to others."
iii. *Logic driven*: "It does not harm me but is of great help to another person. Why not?"
iv. *Self-esteem*: "I feel good after the donation. I like that afterglow."
v. *Sympathy*: "I get emotional when I read about the patients' plight. I want to help."
vi. *Past experiences*: "I am a regular blood donor. I thought I could donate my eyes too."
vii. *Business motive*: "S/he needs my organ. I need her/his money. Why not make a deal?"

The last one is mercenary in character and is best avoided; unfortunately, it may be the commonest motive in India for organ donation. The other six desirable motives could be facilitated if the treating doctor establishes very good rapport with terminally ill cases and explores the possible strategy to persuade them to donate their eyes at least. Without a good rapport, approaching the patient very late or the relatives after the patient dies is of little use.

Prospective donors go through the following steps before committing themselves:

Personal values → empathy arousal → involvement → attitude towards donation → action. You have to facilitate their thought process along this path before achieving results.

ADVANCED SKILLS OF PERSUASION

Mental Judo

When faced by an opposing force, whether physical or mental, you have three choices: fight, flight or judo. Fighting is exemplified by, "When you provoke me, I will provoke you back." Flight is exemplified by, "When you provoke me, I will go away from you." Judo is to say, "When you provoke me, I shall use your energy to guide you to better solutions."

Mental judo is a technique of disarming or redirecting the opponent's force without seeming to offer resistance. It is analogous to judo, the gentle martial art of self-defense, which allows you to defend yourself without inflicting harm on your opponent. It is a quick way of dealing with stalls and objections. As in judo, the smaller person: here the health professional —helps the larger one; here the VIP (Very Important Patient)—land on the mat by force of his or her own weight.

An example: Suppose a patient tells you, "I have been brought here by well meaning friends. I have always consulted Dr X for several years, and he has seen me through difficult times. Our family is loyal to him and will continue to consult him." You may reply harshly (*fight*), refuse to proceed with the consultation (*flight*) or use mental judo.

Using mental judo techniques, you tell him, "Sure. I totally agree with you on the importance of loyalty in doctor-patient relationship. Some day, I hope to earn the same kind of loyalty from you. Now, when we are on loyalty, don't you agree that loyalty to do the best for your own health is even more important? So, suppose I can devise a treatment that would improve the quality of your life and reduce your medical bill, would you agree that loyalty to your own health and well-being comes first?"

Of the myriad of ways of dealing with objections, the mental judo technique of redirecting or refocusing is the most agreeable and persuasive for both the patient and the professional. It is like a sleight of mind. In the example cited above, you not only agree with the patient on loyalty, but also reinforce him/her, making you seem totally non-threatening. Now, you use the very objection (loyalty to doctor) s/he is making and alert him/her to alternatives—loyalty to own health care—that make even better sense. This literally enables you to refocus whatever your patient is stuck on and redirect his/her priorities.

Practising Mental Judo

The beauty of mental judo is that it is usually a win-win situation. It makes both players—the doctor and the patient, feel like winners by preserving rapport in the relationship, by enhancing good feelings and finally, by redirecting the patient to better options, all in an atmosphere devoid of hassle. The professional is truly serving the patient while maintaining control of the emotional climate.

Another example: In 1999, a politician's son got a severe neuroparalytic reaction after rabies prophylaxis, and was on ventilator. He was in coma and the father had the irrational but firm belief that if I took over the management of the case, his comatose son would recover.

Rational arguments did not help. Finally, he blurted out, "Doctor, even if he dies, it does not matter; I want you to treat him." Then I replied softly, "If he were my son, I would rather pray for his recovery than keep insisting that a particular doctor should treat him regardless of the outcome." The politician was sullen and realized his folly brought about by a king-sized ego. He became a changed man and thereafter, maintained a good rapport with all the staff.

Taking the Initiative

Many professionals get angry or upset if a patient overtly or covertly suggests taking a second opinion and say, "If you do not have faith in me, change your doctor." This makes the patient feel guilty but does not address his/her concerns.

You can respond by saying something like this: "Thanks for raising this point. I encourage patients to check with other consultants. In fact, I consult my colleagues quite often to check if my decisions in some complex cases are OK. I will be pleased to give you their names as references. You can consult one of them."

In this example, by first agreeing with the need for a second opinion, we remove any negative thoughts that the patient might have had. We then help them in getting a second consultant's advice before taking a decision. This is a win-win option: The patient gets what s/he wants and you get your colleagues approval.

Refocusing Patient's Sense of Reality

One of my patients was a school teacher who consumed alcohol in excess and all previous attempts at controlling his drinking habits were in vain. Once, he presented with early autonomic neuropathy. I asked him, "*What will happen if* the nervous system worsens and you lose control of your bladder and bowels?" That really shook him in to accepting that he had a drinking problem, enlisting in de-addiction group and getting rid of the habit.

"What will happen if" is one of many refocusing techniques that can cause a patient to alter his/her perspective for reality. "What will happen if" specifically makes him/her reflect on the possible consequences of his/her decision. It makes them focus on the future and the outcome rather than be bogged down in procedural details. In this internet age of instant gratification, this approach has wide applications.

Another refocusing technique is to use "Just suppose." It sounds particularly comfortable to your patient's ears, because it feels so non-threatening.

An elderly diabetic had secondary sulfonylurea failure but persistently refused to consider insulin injections as an option. He used to say, "I would rather die early than take daily shots." Later, he developed diabetic amyotrophy, a reversible form of neuropathy. I asked him, "*Just suppose* that insulin injections can get you back on your feet in 4 to 6 weeks; would you accept a daily shot in order to get out of that wheel chair?" It worked like magic. He took injections for 6 weeks, regained his muscle power and then offered to continue insulin for life!

"Just suppose" is a multi-pronged tool:

- It seems so harmless that the patient permits himself to discuss it
- The professional expands the patient's thinking and makes him focus on positive reasons for complying with advice
- The patient comes up with the ideas that promote your point of view
- You discover the patient's *hot buttons* (what excites him) and seize opportunity for praising his judgement.

All of us perceive the world through a filter of past experiences and psychological biases. Many patients (or their relatives) deny themselves the opportunities to get better therapy or to save on costs because of the games they play with their doctors. Mental judo cuts through gamesmanship by re-educating the patient to better options and easier solutions. It diminishes the chance of false issues clouding the patient's perspective.

Ethical Considerations

Mental judo is potent. Its power comes from the fact that it is gentle and innovative. That, in fact, makes it one of the most effective forms of hidden persuasion. The use of mental judo is justified and ethical when the patient truly needs an intervention and when the cost and risk of the intervention is acceptable. Remember that *you manipulate* a patient when the motive is selfish and *you motivate* him/her when the motive is altruistic. The dividing line is at times quite thin!

BIBLIOGRAPHY

1. Articles on Persuation techniques at http://changingminds.org/techniques/general/articles/articles.htm (Accessed September, 2010).
2. Art Siegel, Five star Yes for client satisfaction and approval. www.salesdoctor.com (Accessed November, 1997).
3. Causal Model of persuasion effect. Soc Sci Med. 1990;43:406.
4. Moine D. Defusing the Toughest Objections. www.salesdoctor.com (Accessed May, 1999).
5. Cosnett G. The Art Of Persuasion, www.salesdoctor.com (Accessed May, 1996).
6. Miller RL, Brickman P, Bolen D. Attribution versus persuasion as a means for modifying behavior. Pers Soc Psychol. 1975;31:430-41.
7. Pratkanis AR, Greenwald AG, Leippe MR, Baumgardner MH. In search of reliable persuasion effects: III. The sleeper effect is dead. Long live the sleeper effect. Pers Soc Psychol. 1988;54:203-18.
8. Soames Job RF. Effective and ineffective use of fear in health promotion campaigns. Am J Public Health. 1988;78:163-7.
9. Switzer GE, et al. Understanding donor motivation. Soc Sci Med. 1997;45:137-47.
10. Weeks S. Health education: learning the techniques of persuasion. Prof Care Mother Child. 1995;5:53-5.

PRACTICAL EXERCISES

Simulation Role-play

Part - 1. Initially the experienced clinicians use simulated patients to demonstrate persuasion techniques.

Part - 2. The students pair off and act out dyads with the following objectives:

i. Persuading an alcoholic, a smoker, and a drug abuser to give up the habit.
ii. Persuading an indecisive patient—with a hernia—to decide on surgical option and fix a date.
iii. Persuading a prospect to donate blood.

Part - 3. In the concluding plenary session, debriefing is done and doubts are clarified.

SECTION 2

CLINICAL APPLICATIONS

CHAPTER

10

Reassurance of the Worried Well

> *Worry never robs tomorrow of its sorrow, it only saps today of its joy.*
>
> —Leo Buscaglia

INTRODUCTION

Much of one's anguish in Life arises from the wide gap between one's expectations and reality. For example, one may say, "*I wish I was stronger, more intelligent, and healthier than I am; I am miserable that I am not. Telling me that I am stronger, more intelligent, and healthier than most others is of little comfort to me.*" Patients who are physically well but unhappy with their bodily state form one such group. To manage this form of *avoidable misery*, we need to improve their perception of reality and at the same time, reduce undue expectations.

"Worried well," constitute a large part of medical practice, and comprise of the following:

- Asymptomatic persons who worry that they may have a hidden disease.
- Asymptomatic persons concerned by a clinical or laboratory finding detected during a routine medical examination or screening. 'Normal' label only reassures half of them.
- Patients with medically unexplained symptoms (MUS) whose laboratory tests are 'normal.' Declaring them 'normal' does not allay their anxiety; they need a causal explanation and a label for reassurance.
- Newly diagnosed patients in early asymptomatic phase of chronic diseases like diabetes or hypertension, who worry excessively about the late complications they face.

CURRENT HANDLING OF THE 'WORRIED WELL'

Most doctors assume that explaining to the patients that they are OK is enough to reassure. A survey of 5150 randomly chosen patients who had recently been discharged from hospital found that a worrying 34% had not been told the result of tests (*BMJ* 1994; 309:1542). Based on textbook knowledge, they also assume that patients should feel reassured by a confident pronouncement that no disease has been found. When patients fail to feel reassured and continue to be anxious, a label of *anxiety neurosis* or '*abnormal illness behavior*' may be pinned on them. However, the residual anxiety can impair quality of life and also results 'doctor shopping' and re-investigations, which are a burden on these patients and the healthcare service.

For example, women with chronic pelvic pain report problems with diagnosis, communication with the doctor, lack of information, and inappropriate treatment. There is a sense of increasing loss of control, as repeated visits to the doctor do not produce an understanding of the pain. Women who had one type of problem tended to have others. Women of lower socioeconomic status are more likely to experience these problems.

Patients who are worried about their symptoms may express their concerns, i) explicitly; ii) as clues or cues for mindful physicians to explore, or iii) choose not to reveal that concern at all, and confine only to factual biomedical data. Most of the patients who present with an explicit concern expect the physician to acknowledge and explore their concerns, while the other two groups were comfortable with biomedical talk. Medical explanations would satisfy the third group, but the other two groups would prefer emotional support in addition to the medical talk (Floyd, et al. 2005).

UNDERSTANDING THE 'WORRIED WELL'

Good communication and rapport building can help these patients. We should realise that-

i. Most worried well cases have an anxiety triggering event like a known person taking ill or dying with signs or symptoms similar to their own, or may have seen a panic mongering media report on such signs or symptoms.
ii. An important reason for continuing anxiety may be inadequate patient understanding that abnormal clinical findings (like a murmur) and benign symptoms could occur and persist even though all the tests turn out to be normal.
iii. Skills in recognising non-verbal cues of anxiety and clinical skills in identifying benign clinical findings—like innocent murmurs—should be cultivated to minimize unnecessary referrals.
iv. Obstacles to reassurance relate to ineffective doctor-patient communication, to the patient's past experiences and to social milieu. The patient's "life-world" and the doctor's "medical world" may be totally divergent or incongruent. Both may have to go half the distance to close the communication gap. An example: A patient may worry about his hiccups because of a firm belief that it is a sign of impending death while the doctor tries to reassure him because his blood urea is normal.
v. Because of the hazard of a false positive or inconclusive test result, referral for such tests should be avoided if expert clinical opinion suggests a very low pre-test probability (see "Tar Baby").

Investigative tests may produce positive psychological benefits (also known as Hawthorne effect). For example, one year after attending a neurological clinic for headache, those who received investigative tests at baseline experienced greater improvement in their symptoms. However, informing them of a normal test result may succeed in reassuring only half the patients.

On the other hand, ambiguous or false positive test results may create or reinforce anxiety ("Tar Baby syndrome"). Direct discussion of patients' concerns and follow up are more likely to reassure patients than doing unnecessary tests of low predictive values.

A real life "Tar Baby"

Ms Mary was a 30-year old staff nurse in a hospital. She had 'heart burn' for a long time. She was relieved by antacid gel and dietary changes whenever needed. One day, she decided to get an ECG done just to make sure her heartburn was not a heart problem, but only due to acid reflux. The ECG showed "non-specific T-wave abnormalities."

Mary got alarmed and consulted a cardiologist. He advised a treadmill-exercise-ECG "to rule out ischemic heart disease." That test showed a 'non-specific or borderline abnormality.' She was advised coronary angiography. As this procedure was invasive and carried a slight risk of morbidity, she was in a dilemma - whether to accept the uncertainty or get the test done. She went back to her family doctor for advice. Her family physician, on learning all the details, laughed and said, "Sister Mary! You have got into the tar baby syndrome. Once you get caught in the trap of a false positive result, you have to go along the inevitable cascade of further tests until all the possibilities are ruled out." He counselled her against any further tests and advised her to continue the treatment for heartburn.

(Reproduced from "Trick or Treat" with permission)

The original story of Tar Baby (Uncle Remus Tale)

Brer Rabbit and the Tar Baby: One day Brer Fox got hold of some tar and made a Tar Baby. He put a hat on it and set it in the middle of the road. Then he hid behind a bush to see what would happen. Presently, along came Brer Rabbit. He politely wished the Tar Baby, "Good morning." When it did not respond, he wished it repeatedly. Finally, thinking that the tar baby was being deliberately rude, he punched it in the face and of course, his hand was stuck in the tar. He punched it with the other hand and that hand too was stuck. When he tried kicking it, his legs were stuck. It was then easy for Brer Fox to capture Brer Rabbit.

The lesson is that we should be conversant with false positivity, false negativity, predictive values (positive and negative) and yield rate of various tests we order. We should realise how pre-test probability affects the predictive values of the tests. This is a vital area of knowledge that enables you to convince the worried well -like Mary- from demanding tests of negligible predictive value. The onus is on the doctor, who has the professional competence, to avoid ordering unnecessary tests.

DEALING WITH PATIENTS HAVING 'MEDICALLY UNEXPLAINED SYMPTOMS'

"The natural state of the intelligent human being is one of modified unhappiness."

- (anon)

Globally, studies reveal that 10–40% of patients in primary care present with physical symptoms without any 'organic findings.' In medical specialties such as gynecology, neurology, or gastroenterology, in 30–70% of cases no organic cause for the patients' symptoms can be found. These patients with medically unexplained symptoms (MUS) constitute a significant group in the health care system (Burbaum, et al. 2010).

Patients with MUS as well as their doctors often find that the medical consultations are unsatisfactory and stressful. The patients feel that they are not taken seriously by their doctors and that the reality of their symptoms is being questioned. The doctors, especially if overstrained by the task of attending to MUS cases, harbor a negative attitude towards them. In such instances, both the patients and their physicians may find misunderstandings and mutual doubts during the consultation and describe it with metaphors like 'tug-of-war', 'brain-washing session', etc.

They often talk at cross-purposes regarding the patient's symptoms: while physicians refer to normal physical findings and test results, patients insist on the reality of their own bodily symptoms and pain (I am not imagining it, doctor). The plight of MUS patients in public hospitals is particularly delicate: they are informed that they will be discharged from the hospital -despite persisting symptoms - as "nothing abnormal" has been detected.

Therapeutic-Counselling of Patients with MUS

Psychosomatic Attributions

Psychosomatic attribution is one of the more confrontational tools in therapeutic counselling. It attempts to create a link between the patients' life experiences, their psychosocial stress factors, emotions and their physical ailments. Attribution is often introduced as a preliminary interaction to assess to what extent the patients themselves can notice a psychosomatic link, e.g. "Do you see a link between your fears and the diarrheal episodes?"

Patients' Reactions to Psychosomatic Attributions

Patients' responses to psychosomatic attributions fall into three recurrent patterns. Explicit responses, like in pattern 1, are rare, while subtle patterns like 2 and 3 are more common (Burbaum, et al. 2010).

Pattern 1: The patient accepts the psychosomatic model but rejects it as an explanation for his/her own physical complaints: e.g. "What you say may be true in general but it doesn't apply in my case. I am mentally a strong character."

Pattern 2: The patient takes up a 'back reference' from the psychosomatic attribution referring to a stressful life situation in the past. By doing so, he/she confirms a part of the attribution but not the attribution as a whole: e.g. "When I was a teenager, may be anxiety of 'fitting in' may have caused the symptoms. But now it is different."

Pattern 3: The patient takes up an aspect of the psychosomatic attribution and puts it into the context of his/her own subjective somatic health belief: e.g., "I agree with you that stress can cause GI upset but in my case, it is not mental - it is physical. Stress makes me vulnerable for GI infections."

Anticipatory Resistance

Most patients like to present themselves as healthy and resilient and not vulnerable to psychsomatic illnesses. Such patients often anticipate the medical interview veering towards psychosomatic attributions and resist it because of worries that they may be labelled as mentally ill, hypochondriacs or malingerers. They are often labeled as 'difficult' or 'problem' patients. Many patients go on to receive investigation and interventions, including invasive procedures which are ineffective and expose them to iatrogenic risks and financial burden (Salmon, 2000).

Dealing with Problematic MUS

Current approaches to doctor-patient interaction reflect three broad models: paternalism, mutuality and consumerism. These are ill-fitted to consultations where patients seek treatment for physical symptoms without physical pathology.
Patients' authority derives from:

- Firm belief in the infallibility of their direct sensory experience of their symptoms.
- Their knowledge of carefully collected evidence and alternative explanations for their symptoms (often contrasts with their doctors' judgements which are rated as ill-considered).
- From their perception that doctors deny the reality and legitimacy of their symptoms. One way to mitigate this is the use of diagnostic labels for somatising syndromes which appears to legitimise them.
- Access to sources of information and advice about symptoms and health care other than from their doctors (Doctors are typically consulted only after many other sources of information have been used. Therefore patients' reactions to what doctors say depend on how doctors' advice concurs or conflicts with what they have learned from other sources such as, self-help books, newspaper articles, internet sites and sufferers' support groups all of which claim expertise. By the time patients consult the doctor, the nature of their problems often seems clear to them, leaving the doctor with a very limited role.)
- Surprisingly common perception that doctors are incompetent to manage their unique problem.

SECTION 2

What do Patients with MUS Seek from the Doctor?

The logical assumption is that they consult doctors because they want their symptoms to be treated and removed. However, there is little evidence to support this assumption, in patients with MUS seeking treatment. They seek emotional support or explanation and reassurance as well as legitimization of the sick role.

It is necessary to appreciate that patients with MUS tend to view symptoms as expressions of menacing entities, separate from themselves, e.g. "the backache problem has again returned to trouble me". In facing this threat, patients seem to value doctors who perform one or both of two functions. One is to give a medical label and explain the symptoms in a convincing and reassuring way. The medical label legitimizes the patients' symptoms and suffering and also reassures the patients that their disease is nothing worse. The second is to establish an *alliance* with them against the disease entity. For the alliance it was sufficient that the doctor was felt to have aligned with the patient to cope with the problem.

How Patients' Influence Doctors in the Absence of Pathology

Given the authority that patients MUS feel over their doctors, they use it to influence doctors. This takes the form of "patients' pressure" for prescription or referral. In the absence of objective evidence, the doctor can not quantify or question the patient's symptoms and must rely entirely on the patient to know the symptoms and suffering. Often patients comment, '*Oh Doctor, but you can't know what it's like*' and demand a prescription or a referral.

Doctors' Counter-influence: Negotiating a Management Decision

If after thorough evaluation, the doctor says, 'everything was normal', then the patient can not dispute the conclusion. This leads to a 'tug-of-war' type of consultation in which the patient focuses on the unpleasantness of the symptoms and the psychosocial distress that they caused, while the doctor focuses on the normality of the body. Doctors must be able to counter the patients' influence on their clinical decisions and they must respond professionally to patients' real needs rather than their felt needs (Salmon, 2000).

Some Do's and Don'ts

- Acknowledge the patient's symptoms as valid. Patients with MUS are accustomed to have their symptoms trivialised or totally dismissed, which signal to them that they cannot trust the doctor to solve their problems.
- Explain the nature of illness and ask them to accept it rather than 'doctor shop' for a suitable label.
- Explain illness-disease-sickness-paradox.
  i. *Illness* is what a patient feels - it is a personal label.
  ii. *Diseases* are what doctors diagnose - it is a professional label.
  iii. *Sickness* refers to the social disability because of the illness - it is a social label.

  In most health problems, these three elements will not be equally severe. You should be able to trifurcate a patient's problems into these three categories. Then you will be able to discuss with them meaningfully and with empathy.
- Encourage them to concentrate on coping strategies to minimize the effects of illness on their quality of life.
- Use the prescription pad prudently: Adding one more medication after the dozens they may have already tried further frustrates both patient and physician.
- Be pragmatically cautious: At times, illness precedes overt disease, e.g. pruritus may precede overt lymphoma by several months. Peripheral neuropathy may precede frank diabetes. So, do not give 100% reassurance only to land into credibility problems later. Keep the worried well patients on periodic follow up.
- Always offer a definite appointment. Advising the patients to seek an appointment "if things get worse" is a bad tactic—the symptoms will invariably get worse. It is better to give definite appointments at regular intervals for review of progress (Lipsitt 2006).
- Remember that "*Worried well can also develop diseases.*" Just because a patient has tension headache for many years does not mean that later in life, s/he can not get other diseases that cause headache. It is prudent to tell such chronic *worried-well* to report for a fresh look (so called 'zero-based approach') whenever the symptoms change in character or if new symptoms appear. I have seen several examples of delayed diagnosis such as, a brain tumor missed in a patient with long standing migraine, and diabetes missed in a patient with long standing nocturia due to prostatism.
- Remember that the doctor-patient relationship itself is usually more important than any specific treatment.

UNDULY WORRIED PATIENTS WITH ASYMPTOMATIC CHRONIC PROBLEMS

Some patients with chronic conditions like hypertension or diabetes may be excessively worried about the late complications even at an early stage of the natural history of the disease. A study revealed that type-2 DM patients were unrealistically pessimistic about their risk of developing CHD/stroke. Their estimates of the risk of coronary heart disease (CHD) of stroke were grossly inflated and were based on relative risk (e.g., 10 fold increase in CHD) and odds ratios than the absolute risk (say, 1.6 % per year). Their mood improved after patients were given accurate risk information (Asimakopoulou 2008).

Their anxieties need to be channeled into meticulous self-care of the chronic problems, making the necessary lifestyle changes, to be adherent to the treatment and to be regular in periodic follow up with the doctor. I find that knowledge of natural history of chronic diseases and of medical philosophy are quite useful in guidance-counseling of such patients.

BIBLIOGRAPHY

1. Asimakopoulou KG, Skinner TC, Spimpolo J, Marsh S, Fox C. Unrealistic pessimism about risk of coronary heart disease and stroke in patients with type 2 diabetes. Patient Education and Counseling 2008; 71:95–101
2. Burbaum C, Stresing AM, Fritzsche K, Peter Auer P, Wirsching M, Lucius-Hoene G. Medically unexplained symptoms as a threat to patients' identity? A conversation analysis of patients' reactions to psychosomatic attributions. Patient Education and Counseling. 2010;79: 207-17.
3. Fitzpatrick R, Hopkins A, Harvard-Watts O. Social dimension of healing- a longitudinal study of outcomes of medical management of headaches. Soc Sci Med. 1983;17:501-10.
4. Fitzpatrick R. Editorial: Telling patients there is nothing wrong. BMJ. 1996;313:311-2.
5. Floyd MR, Lang F, McCord RS, and Keener M. Patients with worry: presentation of concerns and expectations for response. Patient Education and Counseling. 2005;57:211-6.
6. Grace VM. Problems of communication, diagnosis, and treatment experienced by women using the New Zealand health services for chronic pelvic pain: a quantitative analysis. Health Care for Women International. 1995;16:521-35.
7. L.A.Rhodes, et al. The power of the visible: The meaning of diagnostic tests in chronic back pain. Soc Sci Med, 1999;48:1189-1203.
8. Lipsitt D R. Characteristics of patient-doctor relationships with somatizing patients. International Congress Series. 2006;1287:374-7.
9. Salmon P. Patients who present physical symptoms in the absence of physical pathology: a challenge to existing models of doctor-patient interaction. Patient Education and Counseling. 2000;39: 105-113.
10. Sethuraman KR. Tar Baby syndrome in trick or treat - a survival guide to health care. March, 2000, Puducherry, Society of EQUIP. (mailto poligar49@gmail.com for availability of the book)

SECTION 2

PRACTICAL EXERCISES

1. The students may form into small groups and discuss case studies of "Worried Well" selected to highlight different aspects of dealing with them. They may try to trifurcate the problems into illness, disease and sickness. In the plenary session, the tutor can discuss how to communicate these observations to real life patients.
2. The students may form into small groups and discuss case studies of "Worried Well" with very low probability of diseases and work out the predictive values to realise how meaningless it is to order screening tests in such situations. In the plenary session, tutor guides the discussion and helps in choosing tactics of dealing with such cases.

CHAPTER

11 Communicating with Parents and Children

Children begin by loving their parents; as they grow older they judge them.

—Oscar Wilde

Children form a large proportion of caseload in primary care and their parents inevitably worry about them. Understanding what parents worry about is important in order to address their anxieties effectively, to convey relevant information and to impart education.

GENDER DIFFERENCES IN PEDIATRIC PRACTICE

Studies show that compared with male colleagues, female pediatricians engage in more social exchange, more encouragement and reassurance, more communication during the physical examination, and more information gathering with children. Male and female pediatricians engage in similar amounts of discussions regarding illness management. Children are more satisfied with pediatricians of the same gender while parents are more satisfied with female pediatricians. Children communicate more with female than with male pediatricians. These findings are similar to communication patterns in adult patients and may influence gender disparities in health care. Efforts at improving the quality of medical care should address gender differences. *Male doctors must be able to incorporate feminine traits during dyads.*

Masculine traits	*Feminine Traits*
Independent	Gentle
Assertive	Understanding
Ambitious	Tender
Individualistic	Compassionate
Competitive sympathetic	

LISTEN TO THE PARENTS

There is evidence that ***parents are more effective than professionals in early diagnosis*** of a child's health problems. Parents are generally confident about recognising whether their child was becoming ill. They use combinations of behavioral and symptomatic clues. They assess it against any deviation from what is normal for a particular child. While they may be certain that their child is not normal, they are uncertain about what is wrong and about significance of the problem. The other issue that most parents worry about is communication difficulties with the doctor. They also are rocked by parental anxiety, sense of lack of control, and bewilderment at what they see as inconsistent prescribing patterns, unhelpful explanations, and opaque decision making.

UNDERSTANDING PARENTS' CONCERNS

There are two contrasting perspectives on the way patients and their parents use and abuse health services. No doubt, children with trivial complaints, undue parental anxiety, and emergency calls make major demands on a busy doctor's time. Nevertheless, we should realise that these calls also make demands on the wellbeing of parents, usually mothers.

Parents' concerns emanate from a keenly felt pressure to protect their child from harm. Three factors are fundamental in shaping the parents concerns and responses, viz., (a) The perceived *threat* posed by an illness, (b) Their personal need to feel in *control* of the situation and (c) Sharing the *burden* with a doctor.

Perceived Threat

Parents are initially *concerned* about non-specific symptoms associated with their child's illness such as, poor eating, disturbed sleeping and not being the usual self. Parents are *more concerned* if their child has discomfort, for example, hurting from earache or sweating from fever. They become *anxious* if they feel their child is suffering, for example, from rigors of hectic fever or from breathlessness.

Personal Control

Most parents have their own ways of coping with responding to a child's illness. The parents want to monitor and maintain control of symptoms to minimize discomfort and reduce the threat of harm. Parents may repeatedly assess their child's temperature and diligently perform cooling procedures. They are often so preoccupied with control of fever because of fear of a rise in temperature that may go out of their control and cause harm.

Parental Pressure to Prescribe

Most parents cope with feelings of helplessness by actively seeking professional help for their child. This is often linked to expectations of an effective remedy. Therefore, disappointment and frustration occur when this is refuted by the doctor as being unnecessary. Awareness of self-limiting nature of most children's illness may not reduce parental pressure to prescribe an unnecessary drug. A prescription seems to represent more than a decision about treatment:

it helps some parents to cope, some to feel in control; it also indicates that their concerns had been taken seriously by the doctor.

Sharing the Burden

The parents feel that if they ignore the symptoms and something happens to the child, they could never forgive themselves (chagrin factor). At the same time, they may hesitate and think, "Am I disturbing the doctor for nothing?" In most instances, once the doctor has had a look at their child, the parents feel unburdened and a lot less anxious.

The "Black Box" of Medical Examination

The parents generally feel excluded from the apparent mystique of professional assessment. An example: A mother suspects 'chest cold' because the child's breath sounds -"chest feels rattly." However, the doctor pronounces the lungs clear despite apparent evidence to the contrary. Parents may hesitate to question the doctor's authority. They may return home either worrying about the child or feeling silly for the imagining a non-existent disease.

Parents will appreciate it a lot if the medical findings and their implications are informed to them thus demystifying medical examination. In the above example of 'rattly chest', the doctor could say that phlegm in the air passages may cause a rattle but does not indicate a lung infection - chest cold- always. That may reassure the mother that her concern -rattly chest- has been taken seriously by the doctor.

Parents need for more information about coping with a child's illness. Advice about symptom management alone may be insufficient. They may seek explanations, which are specific and practical to help them understand these: The likely cause of the illness, how to assess its severity and when to seek professional help.

EMPATHISE WITH THE PARENTS

Patients usually have a rationale for all their actions, although their doctors may deem these actions haphazard, perverse, foolish or irrational. There remains a divergence of view between users and providers of medical services. Decision-making, differential diagnosis, risk assessment, and living with uncertainty are part of medical practice. This is also true for patients and parents of young patients, though the context varies. Parents' *lifeworld* view of being "a good mother" can conflict with professional views of "good" mothering.

We need to give more information and education for parents. "Empowering" patients (and parents) means recognising their and their children's *special expertise on their own bodies, lives, and environments*, as well as getting professionals to relinquish "their monopoly on expert knowledge."

An Example - A 6-year-old girl was thin and had poor eating habits in contrast to her younger sister. The family doctor found her a normal child but this did not reassure her parents. They consulted a busy top pediatrician who diagnosed "primary complex" based on a positive Mantoux test and advised anti TB therapy. The parents could not accept the diagnosis in an active child who had no contact with a case of TB. A round of 'doctor shopping' ensued. Finally, a physician elicited a detailed medical history of the girl and discovered that she had been given BCG vaccination, which easily accounted for the positive Mantoux test.

This reassured the parents. The physician then asked them to record the body temperature of their girl at 6 am and 6 pm daily and monitor her body weight every week for 4 weeks. This gave the parents a sense of control. After 4 weeks, the parents were convinced that their elder child was normal.

In this case, the parents' concerns about thinness and eating habits reflect erroneous beliefs and use of biomedical concepts within a rational framework. Belief about thinness worsening relentlessly and the parental need to control the eating habits of the child may be viewed as logical and congruent with common knowledge. In addition, wrong advice from professionals commonly reinforce treating many such children unnecessarily for 'primary complex.'

Parents' anxieties about primary complex must be interpreted in the light of media coverage and campaigns about TB. The pressure parents experienced may have been intensified by messages such as "knowing the symptoms of early TB could mean the difference between life and death."

This example emphasizes the importance of acknowledging and addressing parents' fears and beliefs if a consultation is to reassure the parents. Labelling such parental behavior as inappropriate will not help to solve the problem. In tackling such problems, the doctor has to devise ways of enabling and empowering the parents by informing and educating them.

PARENTS' INFORMATION NEEDS

- The nature of symptoms and signs
- The nature of illness
- How to gauge the severity of illness
- How doctors assess illness
- When to seek advice
- Information on 'over the counter' medicines and antibiotics
- Learning about other parents' experiences.

VERIFYING PARENTS' UNDERSTANDING

The most effective way to check understanding is to ask your patient and/or parent to *repeat back to you what you have said, for example* by saying, *"I'm not sure how well I explained that, would you mind telling me what you've understood?"* You should also watch for *nonverbal cues* in your patient/parent which might convey good or poor understanding:

Signs indicating good understanding
- Good eye contact
- Asking questions (means still engaged)
- Forward posture (leaning towards you).

Signs indicating poor understanding
- Loss of eye contact
- No questions
- Body turned away, restless.

ENABLING PARENTS (TO MANAGE MINOR AILMENTS)

When the illnesses are classified as minor, intermediate, or serious, the consulting rate for minor illness is the highest, especially for children. For many doctors, the amount of time taken up in managing minor illnesses is a source of frustration. They know that they can do very little to alter the course of the illness and it is hard to see any benefits from these dyads. If patients could be enabled and encouraged to deal with minor illness, their autonomy and confidence in self would be enhanced, and professionals' time could be more effectively deployed to attend to the seriously ill cases.

An example is the British initiative to enable mothers assess their babies using 'Baby Check.' Baby Check is a scoring system using 19 symptoms and signs designed to enable parents -and professionals- to assess the seriousness of illness in babies aged 6 months and under. It grades infantile illness into four levels of severity and suggests when to get medical opinion. Parents have found Baby-Check helpful in reducing anxiety and increasing their confidence in coping with illness and in communicating with doctors.

Simple Messages Enable Parents

A study of parental recall of their child's diagnosis, treatment, and followup instructions after a visit to the emergency department (ED) revealed the following:

- Three-fourths of parents given a single diagnosis stated it correctly; only about half the parents who were given multiple diagnoses were able to correctly state them all.
- If a single medication was prescribed, 30% of parents knew its name, while only 13% knew all names of multiple medications.
- Of those parents given a single medication, about half knew how to administer it, while only 10% knew how to administer multiple medications.
- Similarly, about half of parents given a single appointment knew the date and place of their child's followup, while only one-sixth who were given multiple appointments knew all dates and locations.

These data suggest that despite high parental satisfaction with detailed communication, many parents cannot fully recall their child's diagnosis, treatment and followup, especially when multiple diagnoses, medications, or appointments are given. *Simplify if you wish to enable the parents of a sick child.*

To sum up, information that address parents' concerns may empower them by enhancing personal control and coping mechanisms.

DEALING WITH CHILDREN

The Commission of Health Improvement's 'Children's Voices Project' reported that health professionals do not always use ideal language, give the right amount of information for each individual or check that young people have understood what has been said. Some children and young people object to the use of higher-pitched singsong-type vocalization (coined 'motherese') which was perceived as being 'talked-down' to.

When a Shy Child Does not Speak

At times a child may speak very little during the consultation. Patience and gentle coaxing may draw them out. A child frequently take longer to respond to questions than adults do, so it is important to maintain your posture and gaze towards your patient when awaiting a reply to a question. Looking to the parent during the pause may coax the parent to reply; therefore, avoid this.

Behaviors which will promote the patient involvement include:
- Adopting an open posture (leaning towards child, arms unfolded)
- Establishing eye contact
- Using his/her name
- Waiting patiently for a reply whilst maintaining the same posture/gaze.

Rapport Building Skills Later During the Examination

Being physically examined can provoke anxiety. Effective rapport building early in the consultation will help reduce this anxiety but you may need to take steps to inform and reassure your patient during the examination.

Rapport building skills include:
- *Company* or *privacy* – ask whom your patient would like to have near/leave the room during the examination (if on the couch), and protect him/her from exposure/embarrassment.
- *Distraction*, e.g. "So who *is* your best friend in school?"
- *Praise* (especially for younger children and detailed physical examinations), e.g. "You're good at this!"
- *Explanation* (about the procedure being done), e.g. "It may seem odd but I need to do this because it will tell me....."
- *Reassurance* (especially if the patient seems apprehensive), e.g. "I need to have a look at your tummy but I don't need to look at your privates, so don't worry, OK?"

DEALING WITH A DYING CHILD

> *Consider the lilies of the field whose bloom is brief:- We are as they;Like them, we fade away as doth a leaf.*
>
> - Christina Rossetti

Dying child is one of the most difficult and emotionally taxing medical problems that doctors face. Our hesitancy to actively involve in what appears to be a futile exercise may be misunderstood by the parents as a sign of callousness. The children are very perceptive and may ask if they would die.

Whatever be their age, the children deserve honest answers and explanations. It strengthens their ability to trust. When we do not provide a straightforward answer, they make up their own fantasy explanations, which can be more frightening than any real, honest response we can offer. While we may not want or need to share all the details of a particular situation or issue with a child, try not to leave any big gaps either. When we do, children tend to fill in the blanks themselves, which can generate a good deal of confusion and concern. We have to first convince the parents and get their permission to go ahead and discuss with their child (See 'collusion' in Chapter-15).

Children live for the moment and they are much less anxious or depressed than most adults. A child may cry her heart out during a painful procedure but will be her boisterous self soon enough. I vividly remember a 4-year-old boy with a complex congenital cyanotic heart disease who used to get short spells of intense dyspnea. Once he felt better, he used to run to the adult cardiac ward where patients were morose, anxious or depressed about their future. The boy used to nonchalantly tell them, "I have 7 holes in my heart—do you know that? Nobody can dare touch my heart except the doctors here." and open his shirt to thrust his chest forward. He was a pet in the adult ward and brought a lot of cheer and hope to all.

Most children accept their life for what it is and truly live for the moment. If you have a good rapport with them, you can give honest opinion and they will take it.

Be Patient

Often it takes a lot of cajoling before a young patient gives his/her story out. As adults, we are tempted to finish the child's sentence, filling in words and phrases in an effort to hear the point sooner. Try to resist this impulse. By listening patiently, we allow the children to think at their own pace and we are letting them know that they are worthy of our time.

To All Doctors, Everywhere (Voice of Children)

To you, we are room numbers, symptoms, diagnoses, charts. We're a group of scientific names that describe why we have unwillingly entered your lives. We are an inconvenient page at two in the morning, a nosebleed on your clean lab coat, a procedure scheduled in for surgery tomorrow morning. Sometimes we interrupt you in your leisure time, and sometimes we mean that you spend less time with your kids.

To you, we are work. Your job. To us, we are so much more.

We have names of our own. Our own loves, and fears, and hopes and dreams and personal tragedies. We are someone's daughter, someone's son, grandchild, cousin, and sibling. But because of circumstances out of our control, we put our lives in your hands.

Please, never lose sight of the faith and trust we put in you. And, as we try to humanize our inhuman situations, please help us. We're not very good at this yet, we're still learning. Sometimes we're cowards. Sometimes, we 're brave. Sometimes, we throw tantrums and sometimes, you may see us cry.

We are giving you a great gift - we trust you with our lives. And, in return, we are hoping and praying that you'll be able to give us the greatest gift of all—our lives back. We thank you for that.

(Web source - Joan Fleitas, Fairfield University, USA)

Dealing with the Family of a Dying Child

Whenever there is a very sick child, the family has emotional swings from hope to despair, feelings and tension run high, and the parents, who are no longer in control, are being tested to their limit. The parents require moral support, help and encouragement to cope with the treatment, which is often unpleasant and distressing for the child and the family alike.

A family practitioner should be able to detect and refer a seriously ill child for specialist treatment when it becomes clear that this is not a minor childhood ailment. Even when the child is at a specialist treatment center, the family doctor has further roles and responsibilities.

Be the Constant Factor

In a strange and often frightening health care facility, the family doctor is the one constant factor. He or she knows the family, as a whole, better than any other professional does. The family doctor was there before the child fell ill and will continue to take care of the family after the treatment is finished, regardless of the outcome. The doctor's continued contact with the family, during the crisis period, can be of help and a source of reassurance to them.

Be Supportive

When faced with such crises, even parents, who are usually sensible, may show maladaptive behavior patterns. They may fail to contact their family physician although it may help them gain support and empathy. Though the clinical care of the child is with the specialists, the family physician may take the initiative to call the family and offer any support throughout the illness.

Promote Good Communication

Poor communication is the root of many problems and effective communication among all the essential players is vital in this situation. If the parents are asked to write down any questions about their child's health care that they wish to discuss, it will make it easier for parents to focus on their concerns and to request relevant information. During the dyad, use that list to ensure that you have answered all the questions; thereby you can tailor the information you provide to the expressed needs of the parents.

Communication between specialist center and family: Initially, the family needs to be informed about the child's disease, the prognosis, the proposed treatment plan and later on whenever there is a major development, good or bad.

Communication among the center, family and the family doctor: Even after the child has been referred to a treatment center, the parents may seek their family doctor's reassurance or guidance. Mutual agreement should be reached on how regularly the general practitioner should make contact to maintain appropriate involvement. If contact has been maintained throughout the illness, doctor and parents may find it easier to cope with the child's death and its aftermath.

SUMMARY

Pediatric practice may be emotionally very taxing because you have to manage the parents in addition to the patient. You need to adopt a positive attitude in responding to the parental concern of fear of losing the child, their perceived need to be in control and their need to share their burden with you. However taxing these demands may appear to be, the rewards of successfully managing sick children is really worth all your time and effort.

BIBLIOGRAPHY

1. Bernzweig J, Takayama JI, Phibbs C, Lewis C, Pantell RH. Gender differences in physicianpatient communication. Evidence from pediatric visits. Archives of Pediatrics & Adolescent Medicine. 1997;151:586-91.

2. Editorial on "Baby Check initiative". BMJ. 1999: 318; 1711.
3. Grover G. Berkowitz CD. Lewis RJ. Parental recall after a visit to the emergency department. Clinical Pediatrics. 1994;33:194-201.
4. Helen Roberts Editorials Listen to the parents. BMJ. 1996;313:954-5.
5. Howells R, Lopez T. Better communication with children and parents. Paediatrics and Child Health 2008;18:381-5.
6. Joe Kai, Parents' difficulties and information needs in coping with acute illness in preschool children: a qualitative study. BMJ. 1996;313:987-90.
7. Joe Kai. What worries parents when their preschool children are acutely ill, and why: a qualitative study. BMJ. 1996;313:983-6.

PRACTICAL EXERCISES

Assignment: Assign common problems in pediatric practice (short fever, diarrhea, etc.) to small groups of students. Each group will make a parent information chart—using text and graphics—to explain to the parents how to manage these at home. All the charts will be presented to the class and discussed to identify their merits and lacunae.

Role-play: Common situations in pediatrics—acute, trivial, chronic and serious problems—may be selected and students asked to play the role of doctor and patient. The charts made earlier may be used here for giving information. Experienced pediatricians may observe these and suggest better ways of dealing with the situations.

CHAPTER

12

Handling the Elderly

> *Grow old along with me! The best is yet to be,*
> *The last of life for which the first was made.*
>
> —R Browning

The world is graying. Due to reduction in birth rate coupled with increased longevity, major population in most countries will consist of the elderly. All doctors (except pediatricians!) need to learn how to handle the elderly.

EXPECTATIONS OF THE ELDERLY

The elderly patients, who have saved for a life time, often have enough funds to spare for their health care in old age and will not mind spending for the kind of care they want. One should learn how to handle them well. Young professionals and the elderly may have a wide generation gap. Most of the values and areas of comfort of the elderly were established a long time ago, when many things were different than they are now. They do not expect the young to go back in time; you are the product of a different time. However, if you want to care for the elderly, then try to meet them halfway. Deal with them in a way that makes them comfortable. The elderly patients will really appreciate that and be your loyal patients.

The following points may help you to understand their needs and deal with them more effectively.

The Elderly are Individuals Too

Try to be creative enough in how you personalize your dealings with them so that they feel that you are actually talking with each of them as an individual, not another 'old patient.'

Never Blame all their Illness on "Old Age"

Every elderly person would know of at least a dozen older persons not having the disease under discussion. Therefore, such "facile explanations" and smooth talking put them off.

They Value the Social Courtesies of the 'Good Old Days'

When the elderly grew up, the society was more formal. When people first met, they called each other Mr and Mrs rather than using first names. Times have changed, but the elderly are more comfortable with people who treat them and their milieu with respect:

- Do not try to become too familiar too fast. Let them set the tone, and read their words and body language.
- Avoid interrupting them while they are speaking, even if you know what they are going to say.
- Do not use slang or profanity; in the orient, addressing them as "uncle" or "aunt" is preferable to calling them as "grandpa" or "granny".
- Subtle things mean more to them. You will really annoy them if you have poor bedside manners.
- Dress like a health professional. Clean, pressed clothes and shiny shoes make them believe that you have a sense of quality that may be reflected in your service and care.
- Do not act as if you think they have Alzheimer's when they pause for a moment to reflect on what you have said. Give them a few vital seconds to respond.
- Do not tell them that they should do something because many other "old people" are doing it.

They are not Easily Impressed by New Technology

You may think that the elderly are old fashioned and that they do not appreciate the value of new technology but that does not mean they are antitechnology. They may not accept the latest technology for its own sake. They have seen too many "state-of-the-art" developments come and go. However, if you will spend a little time and take the trouble to understand the unique aspects of their needs, and convince them that your technology can increase their health or reduce costs, you will have their attention.

Their Expectations are Lower than You Think

The expectations of what can be accomplished are more realistic. So, do not strain yourself trying to convince them that your advice is just the answer to all their problems. Just identify a real problem that needs solving, and show them how your solution will help manage that problem. You will not usually impress them with lavish claims, but you may do so with practical and believable solutions.

They Like to Receive Information in an Orderly Manner

They are more comfortable with communications that have a logical flow from beginning to end, where everything is well connected. You may be comfortable jumping quickly from one topic to another, but they may have a difficult time understanding your point when you do that. So, think a moment before you speak. Fully explain one point about your advice, give them a chance to clarify, and then go on to your next point.

It is Important to Do Exactly What You Say

If you make an appointment with them for a certain time, try to keep it. If you tell them that you would do something, do it. Underpromise and overdeliver. Promise them "Likely discharge from hospital in 10 days", and have them discharged earlier. Since many health professionals are sloppy about keeping their promises, you will really stand out in their mind if you always do at least as much as you promise.

Value is More Important than Cost

The elderly have a long experience and are really *'value buyers'.* They take the long view in any purchasing, considering not only the initial cost but other factors such as expected outcome, service quality, quality of survival and so on.

Elderly Cherish their Relationships

The elderly tend to be very loyal to friends, shops, brands and doctors they have dealt with in the past. They often view the associations as part of their identity. You will not get them to switch to your service just because it is the latest or costs a little less. If you want them to switch, you will have to show them a big enough reason to overcome their sense of loyalty.

PREFERENCES OF THE ELDERLY IN A DYAD

The findings of a study by Greene MG, et al suggest that older patients prefer encounters in which:

- They are questioned about and given an opportunity to talk about their own agenda and concerns
- Physicians provide some structure for the first meeting through their use of questions
- There is physician supportiveness and shared laughter.

In short, the older patients appear to be satisfied with a communication style usually considered characteristic of the traditional model of the physicianpatient relationship (i.e. a warm interpersonal style and physician-generated structure for the visit). They do not prefer a third person during the consultation.

DOCTOR, PATIENT AND CARE-GIVER TRIAD

Elderly patients are often accompanied by a relative or an attendant. Care taking relatives or companions are important during geriatric consultations as they can facilitate communication as well as patient involvement in decision-making (Claymanetal, 2005).

Some of the behaviours which are autonomy-enhancing include the following:

1. Facilitating doctor understanding
   - Clarify or expand history
   - Introduce medical topics
2. Facilitating patient understanding
   - Repeat doctor's explanations
   - Ask doctor questions
3. Facilitating patient involvement
   - Prompt patient to discuss topics
   - Ask patient questions
   - Ask patient to express opinion

On the contrary, at times, the other person may dominate the proceedings and hinder communication with the patient as well as distort patient-involvement in decision-making. Some of the behaviours which are autonomy-detracting include the following:

1. *Controlling the patient's agenda*
   - Answer for the patient
   - Interrupt the patient repeatedly
   - Discuss own health
   - Other controlling behaviours, e.g. belittling patient, insulting patient, companion as expert, "I told you so"
2. *Alliance building*
   - Try to persuade patient to do something doctor wants
   - Try to gain physician agreement for something companion wants

In a study, communication in triadic (doctor-patient-attendant) and dyadic (doctor-patient) medical interviews were compared. The specific content and the scientific quality of interview were not affected by the presence of a third person (Greene, 1994b). However, in triads, older patients—

- *Raised fewer topics* in all content areas (medical, personal, psychosocial, and doctor-patient relationship)
- Were *less responsive* (i.e., the quality of their questioning, informing, and supportiveness was poorer) on patient raised
- Were rated as *less assertive* and *expressive*
- Were less involved in joint decision making and shared laughter
- Were frequently excluded from conversations.

The presence of a third person in the medical encounter changes the interaction dynamics of geriatric interviews and may adversely influence the development of a trusting and effective physician older patient relationship. When ever you notice such problems in a triad, request the third person to stay outside for some time and proceed with a head to head dyad with the elderly patient.

SECTION 2

SUMMARY

In dealing with the elderly, we need to make slight changes in our approach to a dyad or triad. Issues like 'chronic diseases' and 'death and dying' are major problems in geriatric practice. (See relevant chapters for details).

BIBLIOGRAPHY

1. Articles on "The Elderly Customer" in www.salesdoctor.com.
2. Claymanetal ML. Autonomy-related behaviors of patient companions and their effect on decision-making activity in geriatric primary care visits. Social Science and Medicine, 2005;60:1583–91.
3. Greene MG, Adelman RD, Friedmann E, Charon R. Older patient satisfaction with communication during an initial medical encounters. Social Science and Medicine 1994; 38:1279-88.

4. Greene MG, Majerovitz SD, Adelman RD, Rizzo C. The effects of the presence of a third person on the physician older patient medical interview. Journal of the American Geriatrics Society 1994;42:413-9.
5. Koch T, Webb C, Williams AM. Listening to the voices of older patients: An existential-phenomenological approach to quality assurance. Journal of Clinical Nursing 1995; 4:185-93.

PRACTICAL EXERCISE

Standardised Patient–Student Dyad

Elderly patients usually volunteer to let 'young doctors' examine them and learn. Some of the educated elderly can be 'standardised' to give history in a consistent manner. These volunteers can be allotted to students to practice interview skills. The elderly can even give a feedback on individual performances.

CHAPTER

13 Communicating Prognosis, Hope and Risk

Three grand essentials to happiness in this life are something to do, something to love, and something to hope for.

—Joseph Addison

INTRODUCTION

An important part of any clinical consultation deals with communicating prognosis and risks to the patients. Misunderstanding in these areas may result in patient dissatisfaction and possible litigation.

PROGNOSIS

During medical consultations, prognosis or outlook is the first concern of patients and their families. In the Greek and Latin days, while prognosticating, the physicians spoke of *quoad vitam* (life expectancy) and *quoad sanatimem* (quality of life).

Prognostic Information

While listening to prognostic information, the patients generally expect you to cover the "5-Ds" that worry them viz. *disease, discomfort, disability, dissatisfaction and death.* Prognostication is like weather forecasting, i.e. Uncertain but based on sound scientific principles. Prognostication is an analytical process. It is based on the past experiences. It can never be very accurate because of in-built uncertainty, biological variables and risks of therapeutic interventions.

Medical Predictions are Based on Six Groups of Data

Natural history of the disease

Every disease has certain unique characteristics in its natural progression and resolution. These constitute a major factor in prognostication. For example, lobar pneumonia due to Pneumococcus (type 1 or 2), however severe it may be, leaves no residual lesions like lung abscess or bronchiectasis. Therefore, if a patient with this condition can be given reassurance as soon as initial response to antibiotic is apparent.

Time of Presentation

This refers to the point of time in the natural history of the disease at which the patient is situated. This factor is often missed by all except the experienced professionals. For example, if a patient presents to you within minutes of the onset of a stroke with "just a numb thumb," it is imprudent and difficult to predict how far it will deteriorate and extend. Initially, you have to give a guarded prognosis and observe the patient for 24 hours. However, if the same patient had presented with "just a clumsy hand" of 5 days duration, you may confidently give a good prognosis associated with lacunar strokes.

Patient Particulars

Special characteristics of a patient like age, gender, ethnicity, etc. For example, younger patients with stroke usually recover better and faster. Similarly, enteric fever and most exanthematous fevers are more benign in children than in adults.

Indicators of Severity

These are specific features in every disease that indicate severity, e.g. Killip's class in acute myocardial infarction, Glasgow coma scale score after a head injury, etc.

Curability of the Disease

This refers to the amenability of the disease to therapy, availability of safe and effective treatment and the cure rate after treatment. Some positive examples are, purified insulin for type 1 diabetes, Cesarean section for fetal distress and splenectomy for spherocytosis.

Biological Variability

Almost nothing is absolutely certain in biology. So, always make a habit of tempering your predictions with a comment on the unpredictability of most biological events (In Medicine, *Never* means *hardly ever* and *Always* means *most often.*)

Experienced professionals may intuitively consider all these data while announcing the prognosis. The young professionals have to consciously analyze these six groups of data before prognosticating. The language has to be clear, easy to understand and convey "realistic optimism." Avoid brutally frank pronouncements and scaring the patients.

HOPEFULNESS

> *The heart bowed down by weight of woe. To the weakest hope will cling*
>
> —A. Bunn.

Hex Death (Do not Kill Hope)

Hex death is one that follows a ritualized pronouncement of death by a powerful authority, a phenomenon not acknowledged by Western medicine, despite scattered accounts witnessed by reputable observers. Hex was a powerful factor in ancient medicine and witchcraft.

In 1992, case histories of two patients were presented. The first patient, a poorly educated man, who nearly died after a hex was pronounced on him by a local voodoo priest, rapidly recovered after ingenious words and actions by his family physician. The second, who had a diagnosis of metastatic carcinoma of the esophagus (based on an ultrasound scan), wasted away and died believing he was dying of widespread cancer. At autopsy, only a 2-cm nodule of cancer in his liver was found. His cancer was not responsible for his wasting away to death (Meador CK, 1992).

The author knows a prosperous elderly physician who had an asymptomatic 'coin lesion' in his lung. He showed the chest skiagram to his radiologist friend who, without verifying identity or clinical details blurted out, "Poor man; Ca-Lung." The 'victim' wasted away, lost several KGs of body weight and stopped medical practice in anticipation of an early demise. Fortunately for him, another friend of his insisted on taking him through a formal consultation process. The coin lesion was in fact static and turned out to be tuberculous in nature that responded to proper therapy.

These cases raised several intriguing issues. Death from hexing is not limited to ignorant and superstitious tribes. It seems to be a part of some general phenomenon basic to many forms of human communication. Is hex death only a form of human persuasion (or dissuasion)? If we can cause death by what we say or do, then what lesser behavior do we induce in our patients? Can diagnostic labels of serious or life-threatening diseases, whether correct or not, be part of this general phenomenon? What ethical and moral right do we have to pronounce hex like prognostication on trusting patients who seem to have a serious disease?

Hope, Healing and Health

Hope is positively associated with health and healing process. Empirical observations, no doubt rather weak evidences, have revealed the therapeutic potential of hope. Such documentation suggests that hope may—

- Promote healing
- Facilitate coping processes
- Enhance the quality of life.

Medical professionals may perceive kindling of hope to be similar to soothe saying and therefore, be hesitant and uncomfortable in using such tactics while talking to the patients. Nevertheless, one must realize that in the face of uncertainty, there is nothing wrong with hope. Hope is a psychological state and has little to do with biostatistics.

Three Dimensions of Hope

Many consider, hope to be a unidimensional spectrum of feeling varying from extremely hopeful to the extremely hopeless. Hope is better conceptualized in 3-dimensions of personal, situational and interpersonal dimensions.

Personal Dimension

Individual spirit is the dominant component here. It revolves around 'meaning' of the illness - "Why this illness?" "Why me" "Why now?" etc. It is usually based on faith in one's own power to recover or faith in natural or supernatural forces. It is also based on one's coping skills to meet challenging situations and control negative emotions and pessimistic thoughts.

Situational Dimension

Situational dimension refers to the patient's capacity for risk acceptance and it integrates predictability and boldness. For example, a bold patient with a disease, which has predictable cure rate, will be very hopeful of a complete recovery whereas, a timid patient with an unpredictable disease may feel utterly hopeless. One has to fine-tune the reassurances given to these patients so that neither the bold ones end up in "fool's paradise" nor the timid ones unduly pessimistic (see 'personality types' in Chapter 7).

For example, if a patient is unduly bothered about 1: 1000 risk, we have to remind him/her that 999 times out of 1000, patients do well. On the other hand, if a bold patient seems to think of it as being "risk-free," we need to caution him/her that it is not totally risk-free but of low risk.

Interpersonal Dimension

Interpersonal dimension refers to authentic caring. Credibility and comfort factors are major components of authentic caring. A credible doctor and pain-free comfort during therapy gives patient a lot of hope while the reverse-uncomfortable treatment and a doctor of low credibility-make the patient feel hopeless. Outside medical sphere, maintaining social contacts and effective social performance by the patient are signs of hopefulness, especially in chronic diseases.

Enhancing hope—in all its dimensions—can be attempted by helping the patient to—

- Discover his/her faith and possible meaning of the illness (philosophical approach)
- Accept risks and prognosis with realistic optimism
- Ensure authentic caring based on empathy, trust and altruism.

COMMUNICATING RISK

> *I detest life-insurance agents; they always argue that I shall some day die, which is not so!*
>
> —Stephen Leacock

Doctors are poor communicators of risks. In a study by Williams, patients' knowledge regarding the operation, the anesthesia, time spent in the operating theater, amount of postoperative pain, duration of hospital admission and time required to return to normal fitness were assessed. Nursing staff provided most information, *although for the anesthetic, time in theater, return to fitness and pain, more than 60% of patients responded that nobody had provided explanation*. There was a significant correlation between dissatisfaction with information and anxiety.

In another study, out of 100 patients who were given a written information and consent form, only 34 understood the purpose of the form and only one considered it the major source of information. Seventy-five patients could not name any of their drugs, 26 did not know the goal of therapy and only 15 remembered all of four general side effects. Such methods fall short of the requirements of informed consent (Olver et al, 1995).

There is a considerable need to improve information provision, especially for patients in whom anxiety is associated with a desire for further explanation of operative care. We need to understand risk from various perspectives and be able to inform our patients effectively.

Perception of Risk

It is generally assumed that identifying health-related risk factors is easy and straightforward. It is often presumed that once the patients are informed of the health risks engendered by their behavior, rationality will prevail and behavioral modifications would follow. Unfortunately, things are not so simple and the choice is not rational in many cases.

The Language of Risk

Epidemiologists, clinicians, and lay people understand the word *risk* differently:

- An epidemiologist expresses risk in statistical terms as the association between a characteristic and a disease in a defined population.
- A lay person's view is the *subjectivist* interpretation of probability, giving weightage to the context and expectations and by anecdotal observations of events. Tension exists between this view, and the epidemiologist's view, which derives from the *frequentist* interpretation of probability.
- Clinicians try to use *objectivity* and mediate between these two views. They extrapolate epidemiological data derived from a group of cases and take evidence-based decisions in an individual case.

Understanding the following concepts helps in talking about risk.

Hazard

A hazard is a set of circumstances, which may have harmful consequences. It is only a potential risk and does not indicate if it will result in harm to a particular patient, even though we can be certain that adverse events will affect a percentage of those at risk.

Risk

The risk of the adverse event is the probability of a hazard causing such effects. Hazardous behavior like smoking, excessive drinking or unprotected sex carry risk of diseases but there may be other social or self-image benefits, often imagined than real, which keep the person carry on with it. In clinical practice, both diagnostic and therapeutic interventions carry risks as well as benefits.

Threat Perception

Perhaps the most important factor is threat perception, i.e, how an individual patient perceives the hazard. Cigarette smoking is an example wherein the various hazards are well established, yet one-third of adults continue to smoke in spite of knowing all the risks they take. The value of smoking must seem to the individual to be more than the risks of continuing the hazardous habit. *We see things not as they are, but as we are.* (Kant).

Distortions in Risk Perception

Three distortions modify risk perception, viz. using anecdotal evidence, focussing on relative risk instead of absolute risk and only on risks instead of balancing the risks against the benefits.

In the past two decades, media-driven *health scares* have shown that the public can quite rapidly change its behavior, based on anecdotal evidence which is often quite weak. Another trick played on people is to confuse between *relative risk* and *absolute risk*. For example, if relative risk is claimed to be 80% more, and if the absolute risk in normal control is only 0.12%, then the absolute risk of adverse event for the exposed group is only about 0.2%. The latter values do not impress and the media highlight what seems sensational. Thus although the risk of a hazard occurring may be small, individuals may choose not to take even such a small risk and therefore avoid it. A third tactic is to focus on hazards and risks without discussing benefits. Oral contraceptive pills have certain risks but they are all much less than the benefit of avoided pregnancies.

The risk benefit analysis of medical interventions are similar: A patient may have only a 1 in 20 chance of benefit, yet she/he may opt to take that chance and do well. Based on this anecdote, many others may choose the same option and end up with adverse outcome. *Acceptability of risk* is therefore an important factor in decision making. As a care provider, we should elicit the patients' perception of hazards, risks, costs and benefits in order to understand the rationale of patients' choices. To achieve this, information sharing is vital and many misconceptions related to risks, benefits and real costs might have to be cleared to pave the way for rational decisions.

Group vs Individual Risk

Scientific evidence is based on grouped data and statistical analysis of these data, while a clinician has to handle risk-benefit analysis in an individual case. Three basic issues have to be considered:

- How valid and justifiable is it to translate population based risk estimates to individuals?
- Does the risk-benefit analysis meet the patient's real need and is it of relevance to him/her?
- In clinical practice, how can one use a pragmatic approach to communication about risk?

Communication about clinical risks is not straightforward. Estimates of risk derived from populations are often unhelpful in the individual setting (as the subjectivist perspective holds) and that current practice in communicating "evidence based risks" fails to meet individual needs of the patients (Edwards A, 1996).

People often have an "all or nothing" perspective of harm or risk. They may feel, "For me it is not a 20% risk; like risk of pregnancy, it is either 0% or 100%." Therefore, they continue to smoke, or not take any risk with a new drug or an operation, showing that epidemiological estimates of risk are often irrelevant to them. Nobody would disagree that the way we present results to our patients matters, and that individual risk is an important consideration.

Lastly, as with any intervention, citing absolute risk reduction in isolation is meaningless. Discussing the *number needed to treat* (NNT) to save one life or to prevent one episode for a drug or intervention used for primary or secondary prevention gives a better idea to an individual patient regarding the benefit. Knowing that many treatments in other medical and related disciplines have no evidence base is perhaps a more important issue for discussion, including with patients.

Talking to the Patients on Risks

Concepts such as seriousness, avoidability, justifiability, and acceptability are useful while discussing with the patients or their relatives.

Serious-Nonserious

These are words most easily understood by even illiterates when you discuss risks with them. Ascribing labels as unavoidable, acceptable or justifiable will largely depend on the patients' understanding of seriousness of adverse events if they occur. Smoothing talk glossing over serious risks have landed many a professional in consumer courts.

Concept of *normal-abnormal* risks may also be used while discussing seriousness. We tend to accept some risks as 'normal' even when their occurrence is quite high. These are accepted, as "part of life." An example is the high risk of road traffic accidents in India. No one avoids travel by road but grudgingly accept the risk as an inevitable part of modern life. Road travel is a good example to start discussions on anesthetic and operative risks—once in a way, serious accidents occur and unless the patient and relatives are willing to take that, informed consent will have no meaning.

Avoidable-Unavoidable

Whether a risk is avoidable or unavoidable is an important distinction and can radically shift the perception of risk. Avoidable risks allow the patients to exercise their choice. For example, for a patient who needs vaccination against rabies, the risk of neuroparalysis is avoidable if cell-line or chick embryo vaccine is used; but this avoidance costs money as the newer vaccines are more expensive. If the patient understands these cost versus risk-avoidance issues and then decides to take free sample vaccination, then even if an adverse outcome results, she/he can not hold you responsible. Paternalistic decisions either waste the patients' resources or may cause avoidable adverse events and litigation may follow.

Justifiable-Unjustifiable

These are value-loaded words and the patient who ultimately faces the consequences, has to concur with you if the risks are indeed justifiable. In the 90's, in certain mental institutions, many inmates who were unmarried young women were taken up for elective hysterectomy. Although, the relatives had given informed consent for these operations, the society, especially the feminist activists considered it unjustifiable. Paternalism has no role in taking such value-based decisions; you have to adopt the *shared model* of decision making.

Acceptable-Unacceptable

These are again value-laden words and need to be used in a particular context. In general, an unacceptable risk would not be tolerated except for special reasons in special circumstances. For example, the use of an unproved method of treatment may be acceptable as a therapy of last resort. For example, the use of amniocentesis, with its known adverse effects, may be justifiable to detect a particular condition in a fetus. However, if the pregnant mother wishes not to risk any harm to the fetus, she may not consider the procedure acceptable. She may say, "I would keep my fingers crossed and hope for a healthy baby because if amniocentesis causes any harm, I can never accept it." (see "Chagrin factor"). Again paternalism has no role in taking such value-based decisions; you have to adopt the *shared model* of decision making (see Chapter 6).

Quantifying Risks

Two factors in risk-taking behavior are risk-benefit analysis and how patients perceive threat. Some may not wish to take any risks in spite of the possibility of real benefit. Others will take a chance even when the benefit is likely to be low. It depends on the personality of the patient (see "patient personality" in Chapter 7). While talking about quantum of risks, one may use the following grades to stratify them.

Negligible

This would describe an adverse event occurring in less than 1 per million episodes or interventions. Such a risk would be of little concern. This does not mean that the adverse event is unimportant or that the risk can not be reduced even further. Other words like "remote" or "insignificant" may be used here. The word "safe" if used, must be seen to mean negligible risk and not zero-risk. Patient litigation often arises from misunderstanding of the word "safe."

Minimal

This would mean that the risk is in the range of 1 to 10 in a million. The possibility of a risk is thus clearly noted. In macro terms, it might be described as "acceptable," though in individual cases, a decision on acceptability of the risk may vary widely.

Very Low

This would describe a risk of between 1 to 10 in 100,000; many "safe" healthcare interventions belong to this category.

Low

This would relate to a risk of between 1 to 10 in 10,000. Many risks of clinical procedures fit into this category. Other words that might be used to describe the risk include "reasonable," "tolerable," and "small."

Moderate

This would relate to a risk of between 1 in 1000 and 1 in 100. It would cover a wide range of procedures and treatments like major surgical interventions.

High

These would occur at a rate greater than 1 in 100. They might also be described as "frequent," "significant," or "serious." This category might be further subdivided into two: from 1 in 100 to 1 in 10—high—and greater than 1 in 10—very high. Many major experimental interventions may belong to this category. The risks must be conveyed to the patients clearly and not concealed by saying, "Forget about risks. This is the only chance you got."

Unknown Risk

This means that the level of risk is unknown or is not quantifiable. This is common in the developmental stages of a new drug or a procedure or at the beginning of a newly recognized disease, for instance, HIV in 1980's.

Some Examples

Different formats for communicating surgical risks to patients

Surgical colleagues often use the analogy of risks of travel to help the illiterate patients to understand that despite the associated risks, certain actions like travel (and surgery) have to be undertaken. Just as one has faith in the competence of a pilot or a driver, one should have faith in the operating surgeon and his team.

For others who need to know the facts, numerical risk format is simple and adequate in many instances. Vertical bars seem less suitable way to present risks and risk-aversive patients tend to overestimate risk with this format. The presentation of icons is very helpful, but grouped icons might be better than randomly allocated icons because this makes it easier to compare risks. A study (*Timmermansa D et al. 2004*) suggested that patients of the 'high facility and high control' type, who have a higher desire to be involved in decision-making, preferred more complex information than patients of the 'low facility and low control' type, who wanted to be less involved in decision-making. Therefore, the choice of a format to convey risk may be more important for patients with less desire for involvement in the decision making process.

Risk as Bad Omen

Traditional folk, who do not say the word 'snake' at night, believe that if one talks about the dangers and bad things, they will occur. Many of them will stop you from explaining details of what all can go wrong. *Patients also have a right not to know.* Spare them the details of risks; if you are worried about possible litigation, the details could be explained to a close relative who is mature and get that person to sign an informed consent.

Care or Scare?

As a postgraduate student, I knew an elderly man with complete heart block, who used to get several episodes of Stokes-Adams attacks. When medications did not work, he was forcefully informed of the need for pacemaker implantation. When he expressed his inability to afford it, the risks of sudden cardiac death among untreated cases were explained quite explicitly. He then went home saying, "I have fainted hundreds of times till now and I was always certain that I would wake up soon. Now you people have killed my confidence. I am not sure if I shall wake up after my next fainting attack." Unfortunately, minutes later, he had a fatal Stokes-Adams episode at the bus stop outside the hospital and was brought back dead. Did we kill him by killing his hope and confidence? Perhaps so. (see *Hex death* above)

SUMMARY

When you talk to your patients about risks:

- Speak clearly and with compassion; avoid brutal honesty—have some finesse

- Be a partner in decision making, especially in complex decisions. Do not just hand over 'the hot potato' and wait! If patient wants your advice, give your frank opinion without scaring them
- Use language appropriate for the patient; use easy examples and relevant metaphors
- Do not mix up relative risk for absolute risk and odds ratio for 'number-needed to treat'
- Avoid selective use of data; co-ordinate and collaborate with other credible sources
- When discussion moves to "trans-science," i.e. questions asked of science but not answerable by science, say so to the patient; continue in the track of trans-science only if comfortable with medical philosophy.
- If patient seems irrational in his/her choice, inform, educate, counsel and negotiate until you are certain that the patient has been thoughtful in making that decision.

BIBLIOGRAPHY

1. Adelsward V, Sachs L. The meaning of 6.8: numeracy and normality in health information talks. Soc Sci Med. 1996; 43:1179-87.
2. Adrian Edwards Communicating risk. BMJ. 1996; 313:1483.
3. Bloomfield AL. Prognosis (editorial). Arch Int Med. 1956; 97; 267-8.
4. Calman KC, Cancer: science, society and the communication of risk. *BMJ* 1996; 313:799-802.
5. Cohrssen JJ, Covello VT. Risk analysis: a guide to principles and methods for analysing health and environmental risks. Washington: National Technical Information Service, US Department of Commerce. 1989.
6. Dick Madeley. Risks can also be categorised as normal or abnormal. BMJ 1996;313:437-8.
7. John Harrison. Doctors and scientists must be able to communicate degree of risk. BMJ 1996; 312:1037-8.
8. Meador CK. Hex death: voodoo magic or persuasion?. Southern Medical Journal 1992; 85:2447.
9. Nekolaichuk CL, et al. Addressing Hopefulness. Soc Sci Med 1999; 48: 591-605
10. Olver IN, Turrell SJ, Olszewski NA, Willson KJ. Impact of an information and consent form on patients having chemotherapy Medical Journal of Australia 1995;162:823.
11. Sardell AN, Trierweiler SJ. Disclosing the cancer diagnosis. Procedures that influence patient hopefulness. Cancer. 1993;72:3355-65.
12. Timmermansa D, Molewijk B, Stiggelbout A, Kievit J. Different formats for communicating surgical risks to patients and the effect on choice of treatment. Patient Education and Counseling 2004; 54:255-63.
13. Williams OA. Patient knowledge of operative care. Journal of the Royal Society of Medicine. 1993; 86:328-31.

PRACTICAL EXERCISES

Role-play

The tutor has to choose common clinical situations from different disciplines like Medicine, Surgery, obstetrics and pediatrics and allot role-play themes to students. Students pair off and act out a doctor-patient dyad of conveying prognosis, hope and risks. Tutor conducts a plenary session where debriefing is done and any doubt clarified.

Using Different Formats to Explain Risks

The students prepare risk data in different formats like, numeric table, vertical bar, pie chart, iconic chart, and practise on simulated patients to get feedback on quality of communication.

CHAPTER

14

Religion, Faith and Culture in Health Care

I submit that the tension between science and faith should be resolved not in terms either of elimination or duality, but in terms of a synthesis.

- Teilhard de Chardin

INTRODUCTION

Wickenburg consensus (1988) suggested that only 20% of healing at the community level could be ascribed to rational health care. The remainder (80%) could be ascribed to three faith based healing factors-

i. Faith in an inert medicine (placebo effect)
ii. Faith in a doctor or a system of therapy to solve problems (Hawthorne effect)
iii. Faith in nature, God or Oneself (spiritual factor)

It is, therefore, logical to try to include these factors to facilitate early recovery in your patients. Of course, it has to be done within the framework of scientific evidence-based medicine or else one may soon transform into a charlatan or a mere soothsayer.

HANDLING PATIENTS' RELIGIOUS BELIEFS

Here is a list of common interfaces between religion and health care. One should be aware of how religion and faith can facilitate health care processes so that these forces can be taken along with rational medical care.

Faith and Religious Belief

These foster hope and optimism. They have a role in healing process (see above) and on promoting the sense of well being. In fact we find many of the modern day agnostics and atheists, when confronted with uncertainty and self doubt regarding the state of their health, turn into 'worried well' patients; they find if difficult to bounce back to health. I counsel such patients to start believing in one's own spiritual strength or unburden every thing on God and get rid of the 'existential anxiety' that worry them so much.

Religious Commitment

This influences patients to adopt 'good' lifestyle habits. Avoidance of vices and lowering of risk-taking behavior are the positive results of such a commitment. One of my students, who was a chain smoker, got adult varicella complicated by pneumonia. When he feared death, his mother coaxed him to make a commitment to their God that, he will give up smoking if God gave him a new lease of life. He committed himself and then made a dramatic recovery in a couple of days. Of course, the recovery could be just a coincidence but he got rid of a risky behavior thanks to religious commitment.

Worship and Prayer

Studies have documented that these result in catharsis, relaxation, stress-reduction, instillation of hope, and psycho-neurological influences on immune system and endocrine system. These may also help the terminally ill patients face their last days of life with equanimity.

Religious Groups

Such groups provide social and emotional support and help patients to cope with illness with less stress. When one faces a health care problem with uncertain outlook, support groups may help in coping with it.

Doctor as an "Instrument of God"

If patients perceive their doctor as an instrument of God trying to help them recover from illness, then the outcome of treatment is also ascribed to God. This lessens the burden of the doctor after any adverse outcome that may follow treatment.

Handling Superstition and "Benign Magic"

The universe is full of magical things, patiently waiting for our wits to grow sharper. - Eden Phillpotts

However, much you may try to adopt a rationalist approach, 'benign magical thinking' is an integral part of medical practice. Major healing factors are faith-based, viz., placebo effect, Hawthorne effect, and spiritual effect. You need finesse to go along and use these forces for patients' welfare without becoming a charlatan. Accept and incorporate patients' superstition into management plan as far as practicable. For example, if a patient wants to change the date of an *elective surgery* to a more auspicious day, it may be accepted without any reservations.

Similarly, patients often seek change of timing of Cesarean section to avoid the baby being born under a 'bad' -inauspicious- star. Such requests may be dangerous and maladaptive because changing management plan may endanger the patient and the outcome. Then it is ethical on your part to counsel and negotiate with the patient concerned. Creative problem solving helps in such situations. Indians believe in the *power of expatiation* to counter any violation of superstitious beliefs. You can suggest to them to wholeheartedly accept the medical advice and perform suitable expatiation later. This strategy has been called *counter magic*.

Counter magic is by no means confined to the orient. An example from the west: A University professor was certain that she would die during a planned surgery because two of her siblings had died earlier and she would be the third one to close the circle. The belief was based on a superstition in the west that misfortunes occur in a group of three. The counsellor went into the family details and then told her, "Your mother was the first to die, and your two siblings have already closed the circle of misfortune. So don't be afraid." She appreciated his 'sensible logic' and agreed to get operated. Such *counter-magic* often works well to allay the anxiety of patients who are distressed by such beliefs. In fact this tactic is much better than trying to rationalise with them at the time of crisis. Later, when the problem is resolved satisfactorily, you might discuss and laugh about the counter-magic strategy and advise them not to be so superstitious in future.

There are professional hazards of not listening to patients' superstitious beliefs. It has to do with the patient's attitude in case an adverse outcome, say a postoperative complication, results. If you have ignored his/her beliefs and overruled the requests for a change in management, then the patient will keep harping on, "I told you something untoward will happen" and blame you for the predicament. On the other hand, if the same outcome occurs after you have accommodated the superstition, then s/he may say, "It would have been a lot worse and I might have even died. Because we avoided 'it' (the inauspicious time, etc.) I escaped with just a minor complication. Thank heavens for that!"

One person's belief is another person's delusion. These are faith-based beliefs and rational discussions may be of little value in changing their attitude. Therefore, judicious use of placebo effect, Hawthorne effect, benign magic and counter-magic to enhance patients' spirit is good clinical practice. We need to ensure that we do not cross the ethical norms of our profession and end up as mere 'charlatans' who use these faith-based forces for self aggrandizement.

CULTURAL INFLUENCES IN HEALTH CARE

> *Culture is "to know the best that has been said and thought in the world."*
>
> - Mathew Arnold

Cultural differences make a great impact on doctor-patient relationship and on health care decisions. While generalizations are not universally applicable in any population, the cultural characteristics of any society are unique. A doctor who is culture-sensitive in his/her practice finds it easy to make rapport with patients. The cultural characteristics of South Asians and Arabs have been described as examples. Once you develop an eye to perceive cultural uniqueness of a community, it will be easier to adjust your practice in a different community or settings.

South Asians' Cultural Aspects of Health Care

Medical Care and Professionals

South Asians perceive doctor as the authority. They perceive their own role to be passive, respectful and obedient in the doctor's presence. Depending on the level of acculturation, it is customary for the patient to expect the relationship with the provider to be formal. The patient or family will seldom ask questions because it might seem rude. If a Western treatment is at odds with the traditional treatment, the family is likely to ignore the medical advice and stay with tradition. Management of jaundice is a classical example. Even patients with "surgical jaundice" may be treated by traditional methods for a long time.

The doctor is expected to offer tangible solutions and to be confident about proposed treatments or surgery. They think that a competent doctor should not refer to a book. If this is not the case, the South Asian patient may conclude that the doctor lacks skill and may refuse to follow the medical advice. Most South Asians are not accustomed to being informed of every negative aspect of a prescribed treatment. The uncritical use of Western model of informing patients can lead to confusion and fear.

Mental Health

The South Asian attitude towards mental health is complex. An individual's emotional problems bring shame and guilt to the family, preventing any family member from reporting such problems to others outside the family. In some rural communities, mental problems are seen as a result of spirit possession. Exorcism is the treatment for severe cases. Because of their ability to hear voices, a few schizophrenics, especially those with family support, may even end up as "God-persons".

Hospitalization

Surgical procedures are often viewed as threatening and serious. The patient's family needs to be consulted if hospitalization is needed. The patient and family need detailed information about treatments and the length of hospital stay. Although blood transfusions, bone marrow or organ transplants are acceptable to most South Asians, organ donations are seldom approved because of religious implications.

Hospitals should be aware of religious practices involving the wearing of sacred symbols. Such symbols should not be cut or removed without the patient's or family's permission. Examples are: a sacred thread worn by Hindu men of forward community; a Sikh man's bracelet and kirpan (a type of sword); and 33 beads worn by Muslims around the neck or wrist. Strictly observant Sikh men do not cut their hair. If it must be cut, the need must be explained fully to both patient and family.

Gender and Privacy

South Asians prefer to have health professionals of the same gender. This is especially true for procedures or exams involving a patient's private parts, such as pelvic or rectal exams and catheterization. Personal hygiene is a delicate subject. South Asian customs are very different from Western ones. Hospital staff should be aware that bathing in a tub is considered unclean; most South Asians prefer a shower.

Maternal and Child Health

Pregnancy is often the first encounter a woman has with the hospital. Women of the extended family attend to the nurturing rituals and special food requirements of the pregnant woman. Most traditional South Asian men are unfamiliar with these rituals. Women seldom attend childbirth classes. The Western practice of involving the father in the delivery room is unheard of in traditional South Asian families.

Cultural Orientation

i. Because the patient or family will seldom ask questions, doctors should avoid prolonged exchanges with the patient.
ii. Since patients look for tangible solutions, providers should avoid suggestions or treatments that are ambiguous.
iii. In explaining a procedure, providers should balance discussion of the risks with realistic assurances.
iv. If hospitalisation is necessary, family members must be consulted and they must approve. Doctors should give family members and the patient a detailed description of the length of stay, recommended tests and treatments. Family members should be told that they might bring ethnic foods to replace or supplement the patient's hospital meals.
v. The provider should share information about the patient's diagnosis only with the family, not the patient, unless the patient is Westernized or autonomous.
vi. Medical personnel should be aware of religious practices and personal hygiene customs that are different from Western ones.

Arab Culture (Applies to Several other Traditional Muslim Families)

Traditional Healing

An individual who becomes sick will turn first to family members, especially elders, for support, comfort and advice. They may recommend safe, simple home remedies, many of which are encouraged by health professionals. Some examples are:

- Rest in bed under heavy covers to keep warm. It is believed that keeping the body warm will bring rapid recovery from such illnesses as measles.
- Drink plenty of fluids, such as lemonade, soup and herb teas, to relieve abdominal pain and flu.
- Use cold compresses and cold baths to alleviate fever.
- Consume sugar, fresh citrus fruit, honey and maple syrup to ease a sore throat.
- Drink a small amount of hard liquor to alleviate abdominal pain.
- Drink boiled grain water to help remove kidney stones.
- Use bleeding to lower blood pressure.
- Use burning of the body part with hot metal to reduce sciatic pain and gastric pain.
- Bandage the head with a cotton cloth to alleviate headache.
- To treat muscle or back pain, massage in warm soapy water, then rub with oil and wrap in cloth for warmth.
- Use cupping to alleviate back pain and bronchitis.
- Wrap a newborn with several blankets to straighten the backbone.

A few Arabs still practice folk remedies that comfort patients and their families. For example, some people wear amulets for protection against the evil eye or will burn incense to keep the evil eye away from the sick. (The evil eye is believed to be invoked when a person or a family evokes jealousy in others, prompting the eyes of others to inflict harm to that person or family.) In addition, prayers and reading from Al Quran or the Bible help give comfort to patients and family members and enhance the patient's recovery. Many of these are used in India too.

Modern Medical Care

Arab culture and Islamic religion emphasize maintaining good health, especially through personal hygiene practices and a healthy diet. Arabs place a high value in modern Western medicine and have confidence in the medical profession. A patient and family will not wait long to seek professional help. One or more family member will accompany the patient to a medical appointment and stay with him/her to help answer questions about the patient's health.

In Arab countries, patients are told only the good news about their disease. In severe cases, the doctors generally report the seriousness of the illness and its likely consequences to a selected family member. Patients are usually anxious to receive a medication as soon as possible. They will listen carefully to the doctor's advice, explanations and warnings, and will follow the directions carefully. Some patients may argue about lab testing, X-rays and medication but in the end will accept the doctor's orders.

However, once symptoms have improved, many patients will stop taking the prescribed medication or will not return for a scheduled follow-up appointment.

Maternal and Child Health

Arabs in general do not approve having an abortion. Most Arabs consider childbirth to be a concern only for the women in the family. A woman in labor is usually surrounded by female relatives and friends. Fathers are not admitted to the labor room. Midwives play an important role in prenatal care, delivery and post-delivery consultation; they are held in high regard in society and in the medical profession. Arab women prefer to breastfeed their newborns.

Social Customs

When a patient is admitted to the hospital, it is a social obligation for friends and family to visit and bring presents such as flowers or eatables. It is common for recovering patients to give gifts to their doctors—and the other staff—as a sign of appreciation. Some may invite them to their homes or write a thank-you letter in the local newspaper.

Death

Arabs ascribe recovery from illness to professional help and submission to God's will. Family members do not blame health care providers for the death of their loved one. They consider death to be a destiny decided by God. Family members need to be with the body until it is ready to be removed from the hospital. Muslims prefer to bury the body on the day death occurs.

Cultural Barriers to Health Care

Modern Medical Care

An Arab patient seeing a doctor expects quick relief from pain; s/he also expects to receive a medication on the first visit. Patients like doctors to explain the reasons for not getting medications and for all laboratory testing.

Nurses are perceived as helpers, not health care professionals, and their suggestions and advice are not taken seriously. Doctors may need to explain the nurse's role to the patient. Pregnant women prefer to be seen by midwives. Arabs are not accustomed to the profession of social workers. They rely on their families, other relatives and close friends for support and help.

Gender

Generally, both male and female Arab patients and their children prefer to consult male doctors. However, for pregnancy or gynecological needs, women prefer female doctors. In Arab culture, women are reluctant to discuss these concerns with men.

Privacy

Some Arabs are reluctant to disclose detailed information about themselves and their families to strangers. They tend to give as little information as possible and may not give enough for a proper diagnosis. Being conservative, they may be embarrassed by questions about their sexual relationships and other personal questions. Sexual problems and venereal diseases are difficult for Arab patients to deal with. Women are shy to talk about their private lives and may feel more comfortable with women doctors.

Maternal and Child Health

Since midwives play an important role in prenatal care and childbirth in the Arab world, it is highly recommended that pregnant women be seen by midwives. However, increasingly, many prefer to be seen by female doctors.

Mental Health

Typically, Arab society looks down on the mentally ill. Patients with mental health concerns do not like to share this information with their relatives or friends and are shy of seeking professional help.

Diet

Diet may be an issue for Muslim patients. During Ramadan, many patients resist taking medications or eating during the daytime. Since Muslims do not eat pork, patients may not eat all hospital meals. Some eat only Halal meat (meat from animals slaughtered according to Islamic tradition). Because of shyness, fear of rejection, or lack of knowledge, many Arab patients will not ask for different meals.

Cultural Orientation

- If no medication is given, the doctor should explain why.
- Doctors should explain the reasons for all laboratory testing.
- Doctors may need to take the time to explain the nurse's role to the patient.
- Doctors need to build trust with patients in order to get all the information needed for a proper diagnosis.
- Doctors should take the time to evaluate and discuss conditions of a mentally ill patient.
- It is important for health care providers to ask their patients about their diet, especially if they are to be hospitalized.
- Social workers should ask patients if they have family or friends who can help.

BARRIERS BETWEEN DOCTORS AND IMMIGRANT PATIENTS

In a recent study the following barriers were found between immigrant patients and their physicians:

The physician and the patient may -

- Not share the same linguistic background
- Not share similar values about health and illness
- Not have similar role expectations
- Have prejudices and
- Not speak to each other in an unbiased manner.

Due to these barriers, the transfer of information, the formulation of the diagnosis, and the discussion of treatment options are at stake and the shared decision-making process is impeded (Suurmond J, 2006). European physicians, compared with their Asian colleagues, are generally very direct in their communication with patients. An Afghan patient confided thus: "When Afghan people migrate to the Netherlands, they are soon confronted with the fact that things are said so bluntly to them. That they're being told 'you have cancer' and then they're terrified to death. That's a sad experience. 'So heartless,' they say. You won't tell a patient very clearly that he has cancer. This is first said to a member of the family, preferably to a male member, a wise old man or someone like that. They're going to decide within the family what they're going to do and if they're going to tell the patient or not."

SUMMARY

This chapter highlights the importance of knowing about faith, beliefs and cultural background of your patients so that you can enhance the quality of health care. Quality is after all "to meet and even exceed patient expectations."

BIBLIOGRAPHY

1. Ira SenGupta, "South Asian Culture" for Cross Cultural Health Care Program h PacMed Clinics 1200 12th Avenue South h Seattle, WA 98144. URL http://www.xculture.org/ (accessed on 19-09-2010)
2. JS Levin. Religion and Health. Soc Sci Med. 1996;43:858
3. R.B.Blacher, Benign magical thinking. Persp. Biol. Med. 1996;40:190-8.
4. Raja Atallah, "Arab Culture" for Cross Cultural Health Care Program, PacMed Clinics 1200 12th Avenue South, Seattle, WA 98144. URL http://www.xculture.org/ (accessed on 19-09-2010)
5. Suurmond J, Seeleman C. Shared decision-making in an intercultural context Barriers in the interaction between physicians and immigrant patients. Patient Education and Counseling, 2006; 60:253-9.

PRACTICAL EXERCISES

Cross Cultural Empathy training: use students of different cultural background to share their medical and non-medical beliefs; the students are encouraged to give non-judgemental comments on each other's cultural beliefs to convey empathy and understanding.

CHAPTER

15

Dealing with Patients Having Chronic Diseases

I Seeing much, suffering much, and studying much, are the three pillars of learning.

—Benjamin Disraeli

INTRODUCTION

Chronic illness may be simply stated to be any ongoing illness that does not heal. "Once a diabetic, always a diabetic," and the same is the case in hypertension, epilepsy, arthritis, migraine, etc. People with chronic problems can face lots of pain and distress or have limits and circumstances brought on by the illness or disability. Studies reveal that those who are born with disabilities tend to be better adjusted than people whose disabilities came later in life. A person who goes blind at 15 years may lament, "How can I live without seeing?" whereas a person born blind does not have such fears.

There are three types of chronic illnesses:

i. Those which can be managed well and usually without much discomfort and distress
ii. Illnesses where there is not much to relieve pain and suffering
iii. Others which are progressive, developing new disabilities or eventual death.

Diabetes is a good example of the first type. A diabetic may or may not have symptoms and difficulties, but if properly managed, the personal stress and discomfort can be greatly minimized.

In other chronic illnesses, e.g. severe rheumatoid arthritis, the pain and physical disability can become stressful and debilitating. Effective drugs can have side effects and the pain or deformities can be ever present. Chronic asthma and chronic pain syndromes are other examples.

Thirdly, there are progressive chronic illnesses, for example, AIDS, muscular dystrophy or motor neuron disease. These result in continued deterioration of the patient's health. At different phases of these illnesses, there are new emotions and problems to contend with which can cause tremendous amounts of distress.

ATTITUDES TOWARD PATIENT-EXPERTISE IN CHRONIC ILLNESS

A study (Thorne, et al. 2000) explored doctor-patient relationship in chronic diseases in hospital settings. They report that counterproductive attitudes remain conspicuous throughout the healthcare system and cite seven issues:

Loss of Control Over Self Management

Once the patients were hospitalized, healthcare professionals, who had little understanding of the intricacies of diabetes management of the particular patient, assumed that their interpretations were superior to those of the individual who had successfully self-managed his/her insulin dosage for years. Many individuals with diabetes reported serious conflict with nurses and physicians regarding their insulin dosage until they were back home on self-management.

Control of Information Flow

Discrediting or ridiculing patients' attempt to contribute to management decisions and dismissal of their suggestions were some major flaws in the communication dynamics used by the healthcare professionals to retain information control.

Assumptions of Biomedical Superiority

Patients experienced considerable frustration when their own theories or understandings of what might contribute to their illness were ridiculed by health professionals as they had little appreciation of those aspects of illness beyond the realm of what biomedical science makes rational.

Disease Label than Individual Label

Patients often reported that healthcare professionals treated them as "diseases that are carried by non-persons". Labels such as diabetic, hypertensive, asthmatic, etc. promote such behavior even more. Patients with chronic problems would like to be known as unique individuals who have chronic health problem like diabetes, asthma, etc.

Psychological Labelling of Patient Behavior

A common feature of the chronic illness experience was having one's physical symptoms interpreted as signs of psychological problems. In most cases, there were attempts to discount the patient's interpretations of the seriousness of the symptoms; this tended to produce significant distress for the patients.

A 33 year old woman with insulin dependent diabetes had shortness of breath every time she climbed stairs. She consulted her physician on several occasions, reporting the increasing severity of the symptom. On each occasion, she was told that "it was probably nothing." After 6 months, the young woman had a myocardial infarction.

Assumptions about the Meaning of Non-compliance

When chronic patients attempted to modify their adherence to prescribed regimens in order to live as well as possible, their efforts were typically met with considerable resistance and suspicion by healthcare professionals. Consequently, they learnt to "pretend compliance" with healthcare professionals who they perceive cannot tolerate the idea of their assuming control.

Punitive Gate-keeping

Many of the decisions over which professionals seemed to have absolute control could have significant untoward consequences to patients with chronic diseases. A common experience of those with 'Medically unexplained symptoms' (MUS) is the extreme reluctance of professionals to sign required certificates to grant them sick leave and associated health related benefits.

Punitive gate keeping also includes discharging patients against medical advice and suggesting strongly to them "don't' return to us."

If healthcare professionals are unable to value the expertize of patients with chronic diseases, the spiralling behaviors lead to mutual alienation in chronic care relationships. Moreover, one should keep in mind that the needs of patients and caregivers do not always match. A patient and his/her caregiver may have diametrically opposite views on health care needs. The doctor trying to accommodate such discordant needs may feel like the rope in a 'tug-of-war' game.

A "win-win partnership" can be forged if there is mutual agreement on patient's expertize on his/her own body and its functions and doctor's expertize on the disease that afflicts the patient, and that they would take negotiated joint decisions on managing the chronic problem.

DOCTOR-PATIENT DYAD IN CHRONIC PAIN SYNDROMES

The biomedical model states that pain has organic origin and that it may give rise to emotional sequel such as depression or anxiety. It has been the dominant theory and searching for physical damage has been an important element in the legitimization of pain. Organic causes for chronic pain syndromes can be identified in fewer than 20% of those presenting with low back pain to orthopedic specialists. Therefore, recently sociological (sociogenic) theories of chronic pain have challenged the assumptions of dominant biomedical (biogenic) and psychological (psychogenic) models.

The psychogenic theory proposes a causal role for psychological distress that may include the experience of physical as well as psychological pain and forms the basis of somatoform disorders. Whether the psychological distress is cause or effect is often debatable. Sociogenic theory states that medical failure to legitimize 'non-organic' pain leads to alienation, depression, anxiety, and renewed efforts at legitimization. This process sets up a chronic pain cycle that Williams had described as both "a fountain of hope and a font of despair" (Kenny 2004)

Not Listening to the Other— A "Schismogenic Vicious Circle"

The doctor and the patient start with his/her own agenda that he/she wishes to pursue during the consultation, the former on a biomedical (you are normal) path and the latter on perception-is-reality-path. A struggle often ensues in the dyad to dominate the conversation, often without listening to each other. If this initial discordance is not resolved, the health related complaints cannot be resolved. They are revisited in repetitive 'assertion and counteract' rituals (*schismogenic vicious circle*) until either the doctor or the patient quits the consultation in frustration. (*ibid*)

The Cause and Meaning of the Pain

The next set of complaints concerns the reality of the pain. This implicit question is, "Do you believe that I am in pain? My body hurts. The pain must be physical." Chronic pain patients are very keen on convincing doctors of the physical nature of their pain. The doctors may have difficulty believing their patients. Their implicit message is: "If you are in pain, it cannot be physical pain because I can see or detect nothing." (*ibid*)

The Symmetrical Struggle for Legitimization

Patients who reject the notion that psychological distress underlies their pain are subsequently viewed as 'flawed'; further interactions as to whether the patient is mad or stupid are often implicit and underpins the escalating struggle for legitimacy. An exemplar: *"All the doctors I consult look at me as if I am mad. They just write 'this lady is a nut case' in a politically correct way and pass me onto another colleague."* Chronic pain patients not only want a resolution of their symptoms but also want psychological support from their doctors, which they often fail to provide. (*ibid*)

Mutual De-legitimization

Both patients and doctors resort to typecasting achieved through processes of depersonalization and de-individualization (*All of you are same: hopeless!* etc). Endless referrals are the next rituals. This can continue for a long time without spiralling out of control. For some patients, their chronic pain becomes their career, and a full-time occupation! Others often resort to alternative medicine.

To sum up, the challenge for doctors of Western medicine is to adopt potentially healing interactions with their patients that do not rely on the biogenic model of the visible body or the psychogenic model of invisible pain. Sociogenic model provides a mutually acceptable way to continue with the healing and coping mechanisms. (*ibid*)

A significant part of my patient load has been chronic pain syndromes with normal laboratory findings. I legitimize their symptoms by accepting them *in toto* as reality for them. I explain to them that tests are done to exclude diseases like cancer, TB, etc., and that majority of painful disorders do not have lab proof (e.g. migraine, tension headache, neuralgias, etc); then counsel them on lifestyle changes, coping mechanisms (identify and avoid triggers) and to try medications on trial basis. Yogic exercises help them to reduce dependence on Doctors and face the challenge of chronic pain syndrome.

PATIENT-CENTERED, COLLABORATIVE APPROACH

Patient-centered, collaborative approach is a proven way by which effective communication with patients can be achieved. This refers to the health professional's attention to both the psychosocial and physical needs of the patient, fostering a sense of partnership and positive regard, and facilitating patient's active involvement in decision-making (Moran, et al. 2008). One widely used model proposes six interconnecting components:

i. Exploring the disease and illness experience
ii. Understanding the whole person
iii. Finding common ground regarding management

iv. Incorporating prevention and health promotion,
v. Enhancing the doctor-patient relationship, and
vi. 'Being realistic' about personal limitations and issues such as availability of time and resources.

This is likely to mitigate the problems cited above, which are faced by patients with chronic diseases (see Chapter 19 for more details).

DEALING WITH CANCER

In the past, patients with cancer were often not told the truth about their condition. About 35 years ago, McIntosh advocated that the diagnosis of cancer should not routinely be disclosed. This would be considered unacceptable nowadays. In most Westernized societies, where research over the past two decades has shown that most patients want to be informed about their cancer (Degner, 1997).

Effective communication involves more than mere handing out of information; it requires a process of individually tailored explanation, problem solving and acknowledgement of the patient's feelings. The incidence of *anxiety and depression* a year after a diagnosis of breast cancer was lower in women who felt that they were well informed about their illness and treatment options. Women, who knew more about their disease, were *more optimistic* in their outlook (Fallowfield, 1990; Street, et al. 1995).

Patients' Perspectives When Faced with Cancer

A diagnosis of cancer is always traumatic; the patient is suddenly confronted with a life-threatening illness, which s/he may often know very little about. Moreover, s/he may be called upon to make tough decisions within a limited time span, and based on little knowledge of the disease and its consequences. Fear and deep shock are usually the predominant responses to this physical and psychological upheaval. Thoughts of death and fear of drastic treatment or mutilating surgery become powerful and inevitably prompt such questions as - "Will I die? What are available treatments? What are the side effects? Why me?" (*vide infra: difficult questions*)

COMMON COMMUNICATION PROBLEMS

Breaking Bad News

Give attention to the environment and the physical comfort of all concerned. Standing in a corridor or a waiting room is unsatisfactory for everyone. Some persons react by having vaso-vagal attack or syncope.

Bad news cannot be "broken gently" but it can be conveyed in a sensitive manner using words appropriate to the receiver and at a pace comfortable to him/her. Many patients are instinctively aware of the seriousness of their problem. An initial question to check the patient's perception of the situation may help to show that the need is to confirm bad news rather than break it; You can also gauge the kind of words to use. Breaking bad news in chronic diseases can be done in steps to avoid overwhelming the patient but this may not be possible in rapidly worsening diseases, say in acute leukemia.

If bad news has to be broken, it should be interactive -use "Do you follow what I am saying?" at every step- and at the patients' pace so that you can stop when they wish to hear no more. Some individuals may not want to hear the whole diagnosis straight away but may be more concerned with "Why me?" or the treatment that is planned.

'SPIKES strategy' for breaking bad news has been proposed (Baile, et al. 2000):

- Setting up interview
- Perception of patient to be assessed
- Invitation for information to be obtained from the patient
- Knowledge and information to be shared
- Emotional reactions of the patient to be handled
- Summary and strategy for future.

If news is conveyed too bluntly, it may lead to denial; so learn euphemisms and polite words used in the locality and use them. However, with some rustic patients, who use crude language, it may be necessary to be blunt or else the message may not sink in. There is always some level of shock after hearing a bad news, so allow adequate time before attempting to resume the dyad. Rustic women may go on to ritualistic mournful singing (monody or dirge - *oppari* in Tamil). If they break down inconsolably, it is better to schedule a follow up dyad than persist with the present one.

Denial

Denial is inability to perceive something in self or in the outside world because it could create anxiety. Denial may be maladaptive when it delays treatment, or adaptive when it is used only to keep one's cool amidst an uncertain disease process or treatment. For example, a patient with unstable angina who denies any problem and refuses therapy is coping by maladaptive denial. However, a similar patient, who keeps his cool in an intensive care unit by telling the staff and his relatives that he is doing fine, is using denial as an adaptive mechanism to reduce his stress levels.

- Denial may be a tenacious coping mechanism
- Relatives may encourage it
- When extreme, may be total denial
- May switch from concern to denial
- Degree of denial may change over time

Denial may be a valid coping mechanism for patients whose mental make up is unable to accept—or not ready to adapt to—the reality of a terminal illness. Seldom is denial complete or persistent. With passage of time, the reality is accepted. It is important to monitor these changing perceptions and to explore inconsistencies. Strong authoritarian figures like elderly teachers, well-respected religious heads, and tough officials may have difficulty in accepting their vulnerability to an illness. Empathize with them rather than chastise for being in the 'fool's paradise'.

Some patients may also believe in the possibility of complete recovery, although this may change as the disease progresses. You can periodically do a 'reality check' by asking the patient if s/he occasionally felt pessimistic about the outcome. Relatives are often relieved if a patient is in denial phase, for this defers the day when painful issues need to be addressed. They may feel that there is still time to face reality while the patient deteriorates.

Eventually, most patients perceive reality and will give clear signs when they are ready to talk. At this time, relatives may collude to keep the truth from the patient. While acknowledging the relatives' concerns, health professionals must work for and with the patient. Mentally competent adults have a right to make their own decisions about health care, and it is unethical to hide the truth from them when they are ready to face it.

COLLUSION

Collusion is most often seen between professionals and relatives but may also occur between professionals. Commonly relatives request the doctor not tell the patient that s/he has cancer. Collusion is usually an act of love and intended to protect another from pain. Most sequences in Indian movies highlight collusion as an acceptable behavior shown by families concerned with the emotional well being of the patients. Colluders will often argue that they know the patient better than the doctor does and that they know "what s/he can take." They may further argue that telling the truth would kill all hope.

You may discuss with them the reasons for such collusion, but it is also important to explain that the patient's information needs must be met. They must be made to realize that once reality has been accepted, hope can be more meaningful and based on short term, achievable goals.

If you explain to the family members of the ultimate emotional costs of collusion (feeling betrayed) they may let you talk to the patient about the disease. You may often find that the patient is fully or partially aware of the disease but is also colluding tacitly and "playing along."

If collusion can be broken, this can enhance the quality of a patient's life and help the patient and relatives to return to a more open relationship. Honest and open discussion allows patients to be reassured about many nagging doubts and concerns and helps them to plan their life and recast hopes and goals.

Steps in Dealing with Collusion

i. Explore reasons (for collusion)
ii. Determine the costs of collusion
iii. Negotiate access to patients and check their understanding of situation
iv. Promise not to give unwanted information
v. Arrange to talk again and see the family together if they expect it.

DIFFICULT QUESTIONS

Once the unpleasant news is understood, the patient may think of the following questions:

- Why me?
- Is there a cure?
- How long do I have?
- Would complementary therapies help?
- What happens at the end? (end of life decisions)

When the reality is accepted, difficult questions, the answers to which are uncertain or lead on to still more bad news, may soon follow. Questions like "How long can I go on?" need to be discussed. A patient may have certain priorities and goals in life and will need to know if they are achievable.

Dealing with Difficult Questions

- Check reason for questions to focus on intellect and thoughts than on emotion and feelings, e.g., ask, "Why do you want to know that?"
- Show empathy and interest in patient's feelings and ideas, e.g., "It is a tough problem for any one to face up to. What are your thoughts now?"
- Empathize with expressed feelings, e.g., "Yes, Life does seems unfair."
- Confirm or elaborate, e.g., "You may be right," or "I am sceptical about any complementary therapy effecting a cure, but if you have faith in it, your quality of life may improve."
- Be ready to admit that you do not know all the answers, e.g. "The uncertainty in outlook may be vexing, but we just have to hope for the best and wait."
- Convey facts on prognosis with "realistic optimism." Remind the patient that average survival is only indicative and not absolute in any individual case. Remember famous persons who have coped with disability and fatal diseases for long periods, e.g. Stephen Hawking, the astrophysicist with motor neuron disease. Cajole the patient to accept the challenge and face up to it.

Many of these questions are rhetorical and the patients may not expect clear-cut answers. They give you a chance to explore feelings and help you to discuss major concerns. Usually, these questions reflect existential anxieties and center on the inner meaning of the current problems. It may also include spiritual issues and questions on God and religion. The thought of impending death may shake earlier convictions about God and values in life. If medical philosophy is not your strong point you may politely withdraw and refer the case to a counsellor or a priest.

MAJOR EMOTIONAL REACTIONS

- *Anger:* Often misdirected towards health professionals
- *Guilt:* Feelings that the illness is a punishment for past sins
- *Blame:* Belief that current situation is fault of others.

Acknowledging the emotion and thereby legitimizing it, showing concern, and remaining calm will usually diffuse the immediate crisis. Such displays of emotion should not be seen as a personal attack.

In dealing with anger, you should try to establish its cause, see if it is justified or not, and where it is focused or not. Empathize with and encourage the patient to realise the true cause of anger rather than transfer the rage on to professionals. If the patient takes your cues, it may cause healthy discharge of feelings and emotions. Anger may be towards a God who has "failed me" or may be self-directed for having persisted with a risk factor like smoking. You may not be able to assuage the guilt feelings or ascribe blame but by exploring such issues with the patient, you may help him/her towards a realistic perspective.

Exceptional patients are stoic and may use humor to cope with life's stresses like the following anecdote:

The patient awoke from the surgery after a major accident, with the doctor standing beside him. He was told that the spinal injury was so severe, not only will he never walk, but also his life was in danger. Several weeks later, the patient's health had stabilized, and the outlook was for a long and healthy life, although it would be in a wheelchair.
He was asked, "How did you escape death?" "It's really quite simple," the patient joked. "How could I 'kick the bucket' with paralysed legs?"

(Based on a true story of Pastor Shafkat Khan -a paraplegic- in Kenya)

OTHER PROBLEMS OF CONVEYING BAD NEWS

i. Doctors are easy targets for patients having difficulty in coming to terms with cancer and the morbidity of treatment—the "*Blame the messenger syndrome*."
ii. However much you try, some patients will never be satisfied. Hostility from such a patient can be a barrier to effective communication and creates a vicious cycle.
iii. Remember that there are also those to whom the word 'cancer' is an automatic death sentence, and once mentioned, no amount of cajoling or reassurance will help.
iv. Patients of low intellect may not make much sense of indirect or euphemistic talk.
v. Those who press you and pester you to know all the facts but suffer a severe collapse when you explain the unpleasant situation. (*False bravado*)

BARRIERS TO DISCUSSING END-OF-LIFE CARE

Patients with chronic or terminal diseases frequently avoid talking to their physicians about end-of-life care. *Physicians are frequently unaware of patient preferences for endoflife care.* Efforts to improve this communication have generally been unsuccessful, suggesting that important barriers to this communication must exist. Barriers to and facilitators of end-of-life communication between patients with AIDS and their primary care clinicians were identified in a study (Curtis, et al. 2000).

The barriers belonged to three categories-

i. Lack of education about end-of-life care (curricular lacuna)
ii. Lack of counselling skills to help address end-of-life concerns (professional lacuna)
iii. System failure in facilitation of patient-clinician communication (health system lacuna)

Clinicians created such barriers by saying: "the patient has not been very sick yet" and "the patient isn't ready to talk about end-of-life care."

Patients created such barriers by saying: "I feel that if I talk about death, it could bring death closer" and "I don't like to talk about the care I want if I get very sick."

The diversity of barriers suggests that communication about end-of-life care must focus on individual needs and must involve counselling interventions and health system changes in addition to education. Clinician barriers are more common and more strongly associated with the avoidance of discussions on end-of-life care. Therefore, clinicians have an important role in improving communication in this area.

SELF TEST FOR DOCTORS DURING DIFFICULT DYADS

In any illness, the doctor and the sufferer are fellow travellers. The Doctor is a 'care-provider' and the patient is a 'co-provider' because, without the patient's trust and compliance, the care will be of no avail. The dyadic process should generate mutual respect, concern, and even comradeship. In fact, *more the complexity of treatment, more humanism is required on the part of the care providers to prevent the patients from feeling dehumanized.* Doctors may find this difficult due to the lack of communication skills teaching. Other factors include—the lack of support to students' feelings when they confront severe suffering, which forces them to defend themselves by dehumanizing the patient, inappropriate teaching of ethics, and the elitism that characterizes undergraduate medical education in most colleges.

The following questions may be used to assess one's own behavior in a dyad:

i. Have I given the patient, and has s/he understood the literal truth about his/her condition, its treatment, and the prognosis? (*Bridging the arousal gap*)
ii. How would I feel if I were in the patient's place? What would I want to know and what would comfort me in this situation? (*Following the ethical norms*)
iii. Am I sharing decision-making power with this patient? Or am I being paternalistic and denying the patient the chance to share the power? (*Bridging the power gap*)

SUMMARY

Every medical professional needs to cultivate skills in conveying unpleasant news to patients and their relatives. Developing sensitivity and empathy to others predicament make it possible to convey bad news effectively. However, emotional costs to the professional may be high; each one has to develop suitable coping mechanisms to unwind and refresh oneself.

BIBLIOGRAPHY

1. Ann Faulkner. ABC of palliative care: Communication with patients, families, and other professionals. BMJ. 1998;316:130-2.
2. Baile WF, Buckman R, Lenzi R, Glober G, Beale EA, Kudelka AP. SPIKES-A six-step protocol for delivering bad news: application to the patient with cancer. Oncologist. 2000;5:302–11.
3. Curtis JR, Patrick DL, Caldwell ES, Collier AC. Barriers to Communication for Patients With Acquired Immunodeficiency Syndrome and Their Primary Care Clinicians. Arch Intern Med. 2000;160: 1690-6.
4. Degner LF, Kristjanson LJ, Bowman D, Sloan JA, Carriere KC, O'Neil J, et al. Information needs and decisional preferences in women with breast cancer. JAMA. 1997;277:1485-92.
5. Fallowfield LJ, Hall A, Maguire GP, Baum M. Psychological outcomes of different treatment policies in women with early breast cancer outside a clinical trial. BMJ. 1990;301:575-80.
6. Geraldine M Leydon, Mary Boulton, Clare Moynihan, Alison Jones, Jean Mossman, Markella Boudioni, Klim McPherson. Cancer patients' information needs and information seeking behaviour: in depth interview study. *BMJ.* 2000;320:909-13.
7. Kai I. Ohi G. Yano E. Kobayashi Y. Miyama T. Niino N. Naka K. Communication between patients and physicians about terminal care: a survey in Japan. Social Science & Medicine. 1993;36:115-9.
8. Kenny DT. Constructions of chronic pain in doctor-patient relationships: bridging the communication chasm. Patient Education and Counseling. 2004;52:297–305.
9. McIntosh J. Patients' awareness and desire for information about diagnosed but undisclosed malignant disease. Lancet. 1976; ii: 300-3.
10. Metcalfe D. Doctors and patients should be fellow travellers. BMJ. 1998;316:1890-3.
11. Moran J, Bekker H, Latchford G. Everyday use of patient-centred, motivational techniques in routine consultations between doctors and patients with diabetes. Patient Education and Counseling. 2008; 73:224-31.

12. Street RL, Voigt B, Geyer Jr C, Manning T, Swanson GP. Increasing patient nvolvement in choosing treatment for early breast cancer. Cancer. 1995;76:2275-85.
13. Thorne SE, Nyhlin KT, Paterson BL. Attitudes toward patient expertise in chronic illness. International Journal of Nursing Studies. 2000;37:303-11.
14. Turner S, Maher EJ, Young T, Young J, Vaughan Hudson G. What are the information priorities for cancer patients involved in treatment decisions? An experienced surrogate study in Hodgkin's disease. Br J Cancer. 1996;73:222-7.

PRACTICAL EXERCISES

Role-play-simulation on giving bad news to

1. A simulated patient with chronic disease and cancer.
2. An acute disease with bad outlook.
3. A relative of a patient who is admitted with massive MI or after a road traffic accident.

Initially an experienced clinician will demonstrate how to communicate in each of these situations. Later the students will practice under observation and improve by corrective feedback.

CHAPTER

16

Dealing with Death and Dying

Afraid? Of whom am I afraid? Not Death for who is He? The porter of my father's lodge,
As much abasheth me.

- Emily Dickinson

INTRODUCTION

We can not know a patient's mind about dying and death unless we elicit his/her opinion. This truth is missed by most doctors when they talk to patients. A Japanese study examined the accuracy of physicians' estimation of their patients' preferences as regards (1) Information about diagnosis and prognosis, (2) The preferred place of death and (3) The therapeutic strategy at terminal stage (life prolongation vs. pain control). The concordance between patients' preferences and physicians' estimation was similar to that expected by chance alone, i.e. only about 50%. We should to be aware of this. We need to know what is in a patient's mind. We have to elicit it from them.

This is one of the most challenging situations faced by medical and nursing staff. In a large hospital where they undergo training, death is a common daily occurrence and after a death, things move on like an assembly line. However, in small health care facilities at community level, things are a lot different. The doctor has to learn to deal with the situation that may be quite difficult or emotionally challenging.

FUTILITY AND THE CRITICALLY ILL PATIENT

Death in hospitalized patients is an orchestrated event as most of the terminally ill can be kept alive with advanced life support. The medical team has to decide if they are prolonging life or merely delaying certification of death.

Futile stage is reached when the treatment -

- Does not offer any realistic chance of survival
- Fails to offer a minimum quality of life or modicum of medical benefit
- Cannot possibly achieve the terminally ill patient's goals.

This has to be discussed with the relatives of the patient to arrive at an agreement before withdrawing any life support measures that are used to keep the patient alive.

DISCUSSING QUALITY OF DEATH CONCERNS

Six elements have recently been shown to be critical in providing a good-quality end-of-life experience, viz., pain and symptom management, clear decision making, preparation for death, completion, contributing to others, and affirmation of the whole person. While discussing death and dying with a patient, you may need to address these concerns to reassure them on quality of death.

i. Pain and its anticipation is the first concern. We need to anticipate those fears and reassure the patient and family that pain can be managed until the very end.
ii. They need clear decisions and honest communication. By clarifying values and preferences, the ever-present uncertainty surrounding disease and death can be better tolerated.
iii. They need to be appreciated as being unique and 'whole persons,' not only as 'diseases' or cases.
iv. The issue of completion is a key to a good death. Completion includes not only faith issues but also life review, resolving conflicts, spending time with family and friends, and saying good-bye.
v. They need to be able to contribute to the well being of others, they feel good before death.
vi. Autonomous (empowered) patients need to understand what they may encounter at the end of life, in order to prepare for the events that precede and follow their deaths. For example, a patient with advanced emphysema may wish to make a "living will" on when to stop the resuscitation attempts.

COMMUNICATION OF NEONATAL DEATH

A German study was conducted to assess the extent of knowledge which mothers had about a previous stillbirth or neonatal death, their satisfaction with the information and advice given them, and their degree of anxiety during a subsequent pregnancy. Over half the women had a confused knowledge of the events surrounding the death, only 29% were satisfied with the information they had received, and nearly 40% became pregnant within 6 months of the death despite medical advice. *Dissatisfaction with the quality of information given by hospital staff, rapid conception despite medical advice to the contrary, and anxiety in a subsequent pregnancy were common after a previous stillbirth or neonatal death* (Crowther, 1995).

DEALING WITH RELATIVES DURING RESUSCITATION

During active resuscitation, the families of critically ill patients are routinely excluded from the resuscitation area. This protects them from observing resuscitation procedures that may cause distress; the presence of emotionally charged relatives may also compromise the performance of the medical team. However, a controlled study found no adverse psychological effects among the relatives who witnessed resuscitation, all of whom were satisfied with their decision to remain with the patient. The findings may not be applicable to rural folk of India who are very expressive and wail loudly in crises.

During resuscitation, warn all relatives at the bedside about the procedures that would be done and suggest to them to leave the room. The relatives, who comply with your suggestion, can be escorted to the waiting area and be periodically informed about the progress of the resuscitation by a member of the unit. Those relatives, who choose to remain at the bedside, should be accompanied by an experienced member of the unit. S/he offers support, provides brief explanation of the resuscitation procedures and ensures that the relatives do not hamper the procedures in any way.

In acute care situations, there is rarely an opportunity to develop a good rapport with the family before delivering the unexpected news of the death of a relative. The time spent with the family during resuscitation creates a rapport between the nursing staff, the team leader, and the relative, which makes the communication about a death easier for the staff.

DEALING WITH THE BEREAVED RELATIVES

Preparation Before Meeting the Relatives

i. Check your facts, especially the name of the deceased and the nearest relative (Father/Spouse). There may be more than one patient with the same name and the bad news should be conveyed to the right persons.
ii. Try to prevent any disturbances (cell-phone, other patients, calls, etc).
iii. Ensure privacy, preferably in a non-clinical area.
iv. Check your appearance. Do not go with a blood stained operating gown.
v. Ensure that the bereaved person is not left alone. Impulsively, some of them may commit deliberate self-harm.
vi. Remember that bereaved relatives are also "your patients" and your responsibility until they leave the hospital.

Talking to the Bereaved

i. Create rapport: Introduce yourself first; put yourself on the same physical level, e.g., stand if they are standing or sit on a similar chair to theirs.
ii. Elicit how much they already know about the events and the outcome.
iii. Be alert to relatives wanting to know if the patient is dead; confirm it using appropriate words. There is no need to beat around the bush and prolong their agony.
iv. If the deceased is suitable for organ harvesting, permission has to be sought from the relatives.
v. Use clear language that conveys sympathy as well as the message.

Anticipate and Handle Common Reactions

i. Profound sorrow and crying
ii. Disbelief: "Are you sure it is not someone else? Is she/he really gone?" etc.
iii. Guilt: "If only I had ..." or "I should have done ..."
iv. Anger: Against the dead (the incorrigible fool drank himself to death), against God, Doctors or any one else connected directly or indirectly with the death.
v. Unpredictable reactions: Total denial, violence against self or others, paranoia, disclosure of family secrets, etc.

Showing the Body of the Diseased

i. Encourage it but without forcing it on unwilling relatives.
ii. Arrange it as soon as possible; even delay of minutes may appear like hours to the relatives and cause much resentment.
iii. Permit relatives to touch or hug the diseased; in India, orthodox persons do not do such acts.
iv. Offer clear explanations for any visible marks and incisions on the body.
v. Be ready to take care of the relatives if they need medical help.

Other Information and Follow Up

You may need to inform the relatives about the following:
i. Written documents like death-certificate, case-summary, etc.
ii. Procedures about clothing and possessions of the deceased.
iii. Details on contact person, any need for follow up, payment of bills, etc.
iv. Embalming and Storage of the body until they can arrange for transport.
v. How to organize transport.

Prepare for Special Problems

Be prepared to face tough situations and retain semblance of control amidst chaos. This needs pre-planning and mock drills that cover the following scenarios:
i. Commotion following sudden and unexpected death.
ii. Scenes of unrest following death by criminal violence or death of a VIP.
iii. Multiple deaths due to disasters.
iv. Media attention causing disruption.

Promoting Organ Donation

European data published in 1996 identified five situations in which inadequate efforts were being made to secure the donation of organs: *donor detection, donor referral, organ maintenance, care of the family, and organ retrieval.*

Many potential donors are not detected and the *major factor is failure to communicate with bereaved families.* The health professionals who deal with such situations need skills in the management of emotions such as anger, fear, sadness, and uncontrollable grief. Then they may be able to guide the relatives to consider organ donation as a way of keeping at least parts of the departed person alive or as a way of showing altruism (see Chapter 9).

Emotional Costs to Professionals

- Counter transference—empathy and support brings you closer to patients' pain and suffering.
- Inadequacy—feeling powerless to solve patients' problems.
- Failure—feelings of professional failure when the case succumbs to the disease.
- Clinical burden—imbalance between work and relaxation.
- Burden—emotional 'burnout' or progressive cynicism.

BIBLIOGRAPHY

1. Cosgrovea JF, Nesbitta ID, Bartley C. Futility and the critically ill adult patient: A framework. Current Anaesthesia & Critical Care. 2006;17:255-62.
2. Crowther ME. Communication following a stillbirth or neonatal death: room for improvement. British Journal of Obstetrics & Gynaecology. 1995;102:952-6.
3. Hofmann JC, et al. Patient preferences for communication with physicians about end-of-life decisions. Annals of Internal Medicine 1997; 127;112.
4. J Morrow. Telling relatives that a family member has died suddenly. Postgrad Med J. 1996; 72:413-8.
5. Robinson SM, Mackenzie-Ross S, Campbell Hewson GL, Egleston CV, Prevost AT. Psychological effect of witnessed resuscitation on bereaved relatives. Lancet. 1998;352: 614-7.

PRACTICAL EXERCISES

Role-play-simulation on giving bad news to:

1. A relative of a patient who had died after a long battle with cancer.
2. A relative of a patient who unexpectedly died of massive MI or road traffic accident.

Initially an experienced clinician will demonstrate how to communicate in each of these situations. Later the students will practice under observation and improve by corrective feedback.

CHAPTER

17 Handling Non-compliance and Deception

O, what a tangled web we weave, When we first practice to deceive!

- W. Scott

Most doctors assume compliance on the part of their patients because 'they are adults and they ought to know what is good for them'. However, for a variety of reasons, most patients do not comply with or adhere to therapeutic advice. Studies have consistently shown that aversion to medicine taking is widespread (Brittena *et al*, 2004). Aversion means the dislike of taking medicines, which may lead to minimisation of drug taking, cutting doses, stopping and non-dispensing of prescriptions. In the medical literature, these latter behaviours are all referred to as non-compliance or non-adherence. Aversion to medicines ranges over a spectrum, from extreme dislike and distrust of medicines to a slight preference for not taking them.

Deception by patients is common in third world and the Orient: many are reluctant to be frank with their doctors and follow a passive Child–Parent relationship. This is not conducive to an open relationship that facilitates shared decision-making. All of us have to be aware of signals of non-compliance and deception, not to accost the patient but to help him/her receive a better health care.

NON-COMPLIANCE

Definition

The failure of the patient to follow precisely the recommendations of the physician or other health care professionals.

Therapy-related factors leading to non-compliance are:

- Length of regimen—the longer the regimen, more is the non-compliance.
- Complexity of regimen—more complex the regimen, less compliant is the patient.
- Type of regimen—*visibly beneficial* or curative regimen promotes compliance while invisibly curative or prophylactic therapy promotes non-compliance.

Non-compliance is not always total. *Variations* in non-compliance include:
- Slip from total compliance
- Consistent and stable partial compliance
- Modifying the treatment regimen by oneself
- Outright non-compliance.

Why Non-compliance Occurs

Why should the patients do the opposite of what they are advised to do? Why are efforts to persuade them often ineffective and counterproductive? Brehm's *Theory of Reactance* attempts to explain why such maladaptive behavior occurs. The theory postulates that each person believes s/he possesses a set of "free behavior" in which s/he could engage with freedom and autonomy. Lifestyle options (mode of living, clothes, habits and addictions) are major components of free behavior. If health care advice poses a threat to any of these free behaviors, the person is aroused into a reactance state that aims at recapturing the freedom and preventing further loss of autonomy.

Reactance may also try to protect the capacity not to do something that they dislike. An example:

A village headman admitted in my ward was asked by a nurse to give a specimen of stools in an empty matchbox. When he had not complied for three days, the nurse asked him once more rather impatiently, to which he replied, "I would rather give you half of my property than do that." The thought of touching fecal matter was so abhorrent to the village headman that he reacted by outright non-compliance.

Freedom to indulge oneself in their favorite activities and a sense of *control* that protects them from over indulgence are two sides of the same coin. Most patients are aware of this 'freedom-control concept' at least instinctively. For example, while talking about their drinking habits, most alcoholics stress their ability to 'hold' drinks (freedom) and know their limits (control).

Reactance may render the prohibited activity more attractive, e.g., a diabetic patient who starts craving for sugar after the diagnosis has been made. The reverse also happens. For example, a diabetic who repeatedly demands 'a vitamin shot' becomes extremely resistant to the idea of taking daily insulin shots (I don't want to be poked daily).

Other factors may also explain non-compliance. For example, the following five reactions may be observed in-patients diagnosed to have chronic diseases like asthma, epilepsy, etc.

i. "Denier" e.g. " I do not have asthma."
ii. "Distancer" e.g. " I have some wheezing but it is not asthma."
iii. "Concealer" e.g. " I may have asthma but I don't want anyone to know."
iv. "Pragmatist" e.g. " I have asthma problems."
v. "Acceptor" e.g. " I am an asthmatic."

Knowing your patients' reaction to a label like epilepsy, asthma, diabetes, hypertension, TB, HIV etc., helps you to fine tune your responses with empathy and correct their misapprehensions. It is likely that the first three types of reactions will contribute to denial and non-compliance.

The notion of *stigma* is useful to understand the impact of giving a disease label as described above. The stigmatizing process transforms and distorts the patient's self image by inserting a new "spoilt identity" which is the medical label pinned on to them, often for life. Concealment of their spoilt identity is a common strategy; even in the West, full disclosure about epilepsy is made only in one-third of marriages, and in India, the figure is far less.

How to Prevent Non-compliance

- Take the patient along using the shared decision making model based on partnership with the patient; enquire about patients' views of medicines.
- If patients say that they do not want to take medicines, explore their reasons, and discuss the benefits as well as the risks of such action. Consider alternative treatments including no medicines.
- Address the life world considerations of the patient while making medical decisions.
- Make regimen simple and individualized. Make the patient responsible for monitoring, e.g. home monitoring of sugar in diabetics, weekly bodyweight monitoring by patients on reducing diet, etc.
- Use counter reactance, e.g. ask smokers why they can not give up smoking to show that they are not enslaved to it anymore.
- Divert patient from freedom to control. Ask an elderly smoker, "Don't you want to be a role model for your grandchildren? Why not retire from smoking."
- Try to avoid stigmatizing labels. Never tell newly diagnosed patients that they have 'epilepsy.' Call it as 'fits' or its vernacular equivalent and explain to them that all animals including humans can have fits; it happens whenever stress, sleeplessness, drugs, etc. lower the threshold for fits. Then it is easy to counsel these patients on preventive measures and drug therapy to increase the threshold for fits. Similarly, never use 'elephantiasis' to label an early case of filarial leg. It is almost cruel.

Two Techniques for Inducing Compliance

Ask an insulin-requiring diabetic with needle-phobia to take insulin injections only for 2 or 3 weeks 'to give pancreas a well deserved rest and time for recovery.' Later, coax the patient to continue the injections. Most cases would agree to do so. This tactic is '*the foot-in-the-door technique*' for inducing compliance. You begin by asking the patient for a minimal favor and, after gaining agreement, advancing to a larger favor (the one desired from the outset).

The rejection-then-retreat technique is the procedural reverse. It requires that you begin by asking the patient for an action unacceptable to him/her and, after being refused, retreat to a smaller favor (the one desired from the outset). Because of the beneficial aspects of patient perception of concessions, the rejection-then-retreat procedure would be superior to the foot-in-the-door procedure.

How to Handle Irrational Moves by a Patient

Elicit doubts and inform and educate about benefits of modern medicine. Two examples in diabetics:

1. A young man with insulin dependant diabetes asked for non-injection therapy and insisted on trying an alternate system if he cannot be treated orally by allopathy. I had to explain to him, "The life expectancy of a person like you in the pre insulin era was only 90 days after the onset of juvenile diabetes. All the other systems were in existence then without influencing the outcome in any way. Insulin is the only way to control the type of

diabetes you have. Complaining at the age of 60 or 70 about late complications of diabetes is possible only if a person can live that long. I would rather put you on insulin and listen to your complaints thirty years later, than let you suffer a bad result within a few months due to neglect."

2. An elderly man with non-insulin dependant diabetes with very high blood sugar values wanted to know if he could start eating bitter gourd to control his sugar and avoid taking pills. I told him that in order to control such high sugar values he might have to take half kg or more of bitter gourd as against half of a tiny tablet costing only a small fraction. Once he considered the cost and convenience, he became totally compliant.

Some cases e.g., nephrotic syndrome, require modern medicine but plan to shift to faith based therapies. I tell them, "If you have as much faith in my advice and in allopathic system, the results will be much better. You will benefit from rational therapy and faith based healing rather than only the latter, which may harm you in the long run." Some get convinced, some others combine modern therapy with faith based healing practices.

DEALING WITH DECEPTIVE PATIENTS

The deception is frustrating. The patient appears to be compliant but then does not adhere to the management plan. Some patients may feel uncomfortable telling you "No" to your face. Some others may have no problem with confrontation at all but may not want to waste their time in explaining their objections to you and having you respond. For them, it is easier to offer no resistance at all and then quietly go off somewhere else for treatment.

Your job is to spot such patients early and deepen the dialogue, even if it means making them a little uncomfortable at first. Experienced professionals develop a sixth sense that can spot signs of non-compliance. You too can develop it.

Common Pitfalls

Mistaking Good Rapport for Compliance

Young professionals often assume that good rapport means good compliance. Nothing could be further from the truth. With most patients, it is easy to make friends without making them follow your advice.

The truth is, the less exclusive your practice, the more likely that your patient consults you for emotional rather than logical reasons. For example, an asthmatic or a diabetic can consult a hundred physicians for advice. The reason for consulting you is based more on personal rapport. However, if your advice were not acceptable to the patient, he/she would quietly go elsewhere. On the other hand, an exclusive plastic surgeon, well known for cosmetic surgery, will get patients more due to a logical need for that service. Those who consult the surgeon are more likely to comply with the advice given even if the surgeon is reticent or rude.

Assuming Compliance in Tacit Patients

Any patient keen on therapy is bound to have some objections to your advice or at least some clarifications to seek. Raising objections like "Why should I do it?" or "Why can't I continue the present regimen?" is a natural part of the process of accepting any advice. If no objections are raised or clarifications sought, then these are warning signs that something is wrong and that you may have a non-compliant patient on hand. It is, therefore, better to raise the objection yourself than remain in fool's paradise.

Mistaking Patients' Appreciation for Compliance

Appreciative comments from most patients are signals of compliance but in the case of *approval seeking* patients, they simply are not. They may not intend to follow your advice and may be extra nice to you because they do not want to upset you and spoil the emotional climate of the dyad. They act "Nice" and then fade away!

You should be able to spot such false signals early and react appropriately. Some of them are:

- The patient does not seek any clarifications and the dyad is not two-way.
- The dyad seems too short to really convince someone.
- The patient makes personal rapport with you, but the dyad does not deal much about the health problem.
- The patient seems a little "too nice," almost like apologizing for something.
- The patient does not raise any of the objections that patients with such a condition usually raise; convincing the patient seems a little too easy.
- If you read body language well, you may detect signs of deception when the patient verbalizes or listens to your advice. (see Non-verbal behavior)

Strategies for Handling Deceptive and Hesitant Patients

Deepen the dialogue from a friendly chat to a professional call

Accept the friendly facade, but try to get to the real issues in case management. You do not have to offend, but you do have to initiate a deeper, more business-like dialogue. In most cases, the patient will respond to this positively. Although the patient seems to resist a more professional dyad, at some level s/he expects you to pursue it.

Making the transition from friendly chat to the more clinical dyad

- For a soft transition, raise a general question about the treatment process: "I want to ask you this. Do you really intend to get treated this way or should it be different?" The response such a general query elicits can be followed up with specific questions in a more clinical way.
- A more direct transition can be made simply by asking for it directly, "Before you leave today, we really have to plan an acceptable treatment plan for you." or "Now listen carefully. There is something new you need to think about." Then move into the clinical details.
- Sometimes the patients may resist formal presentation by saying, "Spare me the details, doctor." In this situation, simply say that you have a set of points that you need to clarify with the patient. You start an interactive conversation based on a series of "Don't you want to know about...?" questions. This tactic is very useful in getting an informed consent for major procedures from reticent patients. If things go wrong afterwards, you will be held responsible for not explaining the risks or costs adequately. If the patient does not want to know, then inform a close relative about the details of outlook.

Make Decision-making Appear Smart

Sometimes hesitant patients are new to the hospital setting and really do not know how to decide but ultimately they will be judged on the merits of their health care decisions. If you are to retain them as your patients, you will have to help them to look good while they accept treatment from you. What you can do is throw out a few tips to your patient on how to be a smart patient. You might suggest, "If I were you, I would consider..." or you might mention some other prominent people in similar situation behave in certain ways that are to their advantage.

I often use this to convince patients who are reluctant to take effective treatment, say paracetamol, because it is simple and inexpensive. I tell them, "Even astronauts take this tablet in their medical kit to the Moon." Similarly, when a stroke patient feels that enough is not being done, I relate to them that whatever was done to "MGR" (the former chief minister of Tamil Nadu) when he had stroke, is being done to him/her.

Get the Patients on Your Side

Elderly dependants, housewives, neglected girl-children are some of the cases who need this approach. If you can convince them that you will try to get approval from their relatives for their treatment, then even the most insecure patient can be won over.

The first thing you have to do is really convince them that they should follow your advice. Then position yourself as a helper who will help your patients get what they are looking for. After you get them on your side, ask, "Is there someone else I have to talk to?" Ask, "Is there anyone else I can meet within your family who can help you to get treated this way?" Of course, the onus will be on you to follow up on these cases and convince their relatives of the need for therapy.

Bring up Objections Yourself

With most patients, this would be a very tricky thing to do. Why would you introduce problems and concerns that may not be on the mind of the patient at this time? The problem with most hesitant patients is that they are not making the decisions. After leaving the clinic, they go to elders in the family and say, "I like to get treated there." The elders may raise objections and you will not be there to deal with them.

What you might do to raise these objections is to say, "Later on, you may have some concerns about the treatment or your relatives may raise some queries in my absence. Let me mention a few of the typical ones that usually come up. If you think that some of those are important to you, I can explain to you further." This way you give the patients an opportunity to choose among the objections without overwhelming them with a whole bunch of reasons why they should not be treated.

Stage a Gentle "Confrontation"

The day patients decide they are leaving you for some other therapy, their behavior towards you changes. Tough patients become thankful; reticent patients become friendly. *The objections are gone, but so are these patients!* If you happen to notice such ominous changes, you could check it out by asking your patients indirectly, say for example, how they plan to cope with the illness during the next month or next year.

While you are talking with such patients, something—subconscious reading of body language—tells you that some patients are not convinced and may not comply with your advice, even though verbally they say they would do so. With experience, you will get this feeling more often (see "Signs of deception").

You can provoke a gentle *tete a tete* by expressing an uncomfortable feeling. You might say, "It is not that I disbelieve you but I am still concerned that—." Here, your concerns should focus on the specifics of the case management that bothers you, such as not getting a firm commitment on a surgical option advised by you.

It is my habit to tell such patients, who have a good rapport but show signs of hesitancy, "I am double checking this with you for my own sake. If you can assure me that you will get treated without fail, then I can sleep peacefully tonight. Otherwise, I will keep on worrying if I let you off without giving proper advice or clearing your lingering doubts."

Finalise the Level of Commitment

Before your patients walk out the door, make sure you understand, in very specific terms, just how committed each patient is. Here are some approaches to find out:

- *Ask for proof.* If the patient was advised to take some injections, verify by questioning, if it has been taken. The proof could be in the form of purchase bills, used medicine containers or even a description of the drug say, the shape of a tablet or its effect as the metallic taste after taking metronidazole.
- *Ask for a dead line.* How much longer will it take before a commitment can be made? Maybe this patient has to meet with the rest of the family. Maybe this patient has to get a second opinion and even a third one. Find out what is the time-scale in the patient's mind. Patients with chronic stable problems like hydrocoele or tooth-decay may take many years to accept treatment.
- *Find a way to continue the dialogue.* Before the patient leaves the room, ask what is next. When does s/he plan to get back to you? Find out whether the patient would like to maintain contact when situation warrants it. If a patient is the vacillating type, you need to maintain some sort of dialogue with this person, even if it has nothing to do with the particular illness that you are treating at present.

Tactics to Adopt When You Lose Patients to Follow Up

You thought you had done a competent job and now you find that your patient has dropped out of therapy. You could react using one or more of the following tactics:

- *Act immediately.* If you are trying to reverse an irrational decision made by a patient or his/her relatives, then the longer a decision stands unquestioned, the more likely it will stand forever. Hours and days count. A decision that has just made can often be reversed. Timing is everything, and you have to get in and see the decision-maker fast.

  This tactic is useful in handling paediatric cases like meningitis or infective endocarditis, which are half way into life saving therapy, and then suddenly the father decides to stop treatment of his child. If you are lax in convincing the decision-maker, it may be too late to save the child.
- *Gather information*: Use any rapport you have to get the details. First of all, you have to find out what happened, what went wrong, who talked to whom, what was said, what information was shared that persuaded your patient to stop treatment.
- *Use friendliness*: "I would like you to come and listen to my suggestions one more time. I could help you to get better by a more effective, less painful, less expensive therapy. What do you say?"

- *Make an emotional appeal*: "I can't believe that you have dropped out! I want to contact someone senior in your family. If you wanted a second opinion, had you checked with me first, I would have gladly given you a proper referral note." This tactic may work well with your patients with chronic diseases who periodically go "doctor-shopping" and then return to you.
  You can be proactive. If they show signs of indifference during a dyad, check with them if you should refer them to any other doctor.
- *Use a more logical approach*: "At least tell me what happened." and then listen very carefully to what did happen. Use this tactic with patients, who are reticent because they feel silly, sad or guilty of discontinuing your care and going of on a doctor-shopping spree.
- *Use guilt*: "I am so surprised! I thought we had a real understanding. I did not imagine that you would go off to someone else without at least telling me first. I would have warned you of this outcome."
  This tactic works well when the patient has opted for a less effective form of therapy because it is more convenient or pleasant but ends up with a poor outcome. Common examples are found among hypertensives, diabetics and asthmatics, who suddenly shift to an alternate system of therapy and present to you later with accelerated hypertension, diabetic ketosis and acute severe asthma respectively.
- *Use intimidation*: "I can't believe you didn't follow my advice. Do you really think it is in the best interests of you and your family to do such a thing? I can't imagine that your relatives don't want you to get the best treatment possible. I don't know how dropping off treatment is going to make you look if you get into any thing serious later."
  Use this tactic only as a last resort and in the best interests of patients when they are irrationally non-compliant, like omitting a life-saving therapy due to whims and fancies. An example is a young married woman with hypothyroidism, who repeatedly defaults in taking T4 therapy despite warnings on adverse effects of non-compliance on reproductive health and on a fetus.
- *Never say, "It is too late."* If you are dealing with a patient who is poor in making commitments, the worst thing you can do is to say it is too late. Then this patient will follow the path of least resistance and continue to be non-compliant. Just assume that it is not too late, cross your fingers and proceed accordingly.
  This tactic may be very useful in managing alcoholics or smokers who may feel, "It is too late anyway; why give up the habit now?" By persistent coaxing, motivation and saying "It is never too late. You can do it even now and find some benefit," I have made several elderly patients give up their addiction.
- *Learn for the next time.* If you lose a case to follow up, learn from it, so that the next round, if there is one, will go more to your favor.

Closure of the dyad with hesitant patients

Treat it like a normal dyad once you have tackled the cause of reticence, hesitancy or non-compliance. Once you get past the patient's wall of resistance and veil of ignorance, get into a more clinical dialogue. Closure of the dyad proceeds very much like a normal one. The trick is to get past the smoke screen to break the wall or remove the veil. That is indeed an art and a science.

BIBLIOGRAPHY

1. Brittena N, Stevenson F, Gafarangac J, Barryd C, Bradley C. The expression of aversion to medicines in general practice consultations. Social Science & Medicine. 2004;59:1495–1503.
2. Cialdini RB. A test of two techniques for inducing verbal, behavioral, and further compliance with a request to give blood. pp 17686. In: Weiss SM, ed. Proceedings of the National Heart and Lung Institute Working Conference on health behavior. Bethesda, NIH, 1975.
3. Fogarty JS. Reactance theory and patient non-compliance. Soc Sci Med. 1997;45:1277-88.
4. Josh Gordon. Excerpts From his Book: Tough Calls, Published 3/31/97 in www.salesdoctor.com.

PRACTICAL EXERCISES

Role-play simulation: Senior staff may do role-plays with simulated patients to show the seven strategies of dealing with deceptive and hesitant patients. The students will observe these with the help of a checklist and discuss their impressions in the plenary session.

SECTION 3

BEYOND COMMUNICATION

CHAPTER

18

Dealing with Patient Dissatisfaction

> *I do not love thee, Doctor Fell: The reason why I cannot tell;But this I know, and know fully well: I do not love thee, Doctor Fell.*
>
> —T. Brown

INTRODUCTION

Routine doctor-patient communication differs between primary care physicians with or without prior malpractice claims. A study by Levinson et al showed that "No-claims physicians" educated the patients about what to expect, laughed and used humor more, and used more facilitation (soliciting patients' opinions, checking understanding, and encouraging patients to talk). It is apparent that promoting patient satisfaction reduces the chance of malpractice claims. One has to also understand various factors that result in patient dissatisfaction and avoid them during dyads.

PERCEIVING PATIENT DISSATISFACTION

A study done in Norway revealed that doctors were able to correctly identify patient satisfaction only in 50% of the consultations. This was no better than "tossing a coin". Doctors with more experience were more accurate in their assessments. Doctors need to cultivate the insight to perceive patients' responses during dyads.

EFFECT OF DOCTOR'S AGE AND GENDER

In studies by Hall et al, patients examined by younger physicians, especially younger female physicians, reported lower ratings of satisfaction. These findings were true for the male and female patients. However, in both studies, the lowest satisfaction in absolute terms was among male patients examined by younger female physicians. The effects were not explained by patient and physician background characteristics or by measured communication during the visit. Gender-related values and expectations influence patients' reactions to the physicians' behavior. It is prudent for young doctors, especially females, to dress formally and display a professional attitude that may be more acceptable to the patients (see 'non-verbal behaviour').

INPATIENT DISSATISFACTION

Delbanco et al studied the patient perception of quality of inpatient care in the United States. One-third of the patients reported that that physician did not care for them during hospitalization. Other problems included:

- Not receiving information about the hospital routine,
- Not being told whom to ask for help,
- Having pain that could have been relieved by more prompt attention, and
- Not being given adequate information and guidance about after-discharge care.

Most patients (95%) preferred to be informed about the important aspects of their care but their preferences for involvement in care varied widely.

In-patient satisfaction is increasingly being measured as an indication of the effectiveness of nursing care. Thomas et al identified eleven nursing care parameters that correlated with patient satisfaction: ***nurses' manner, attentiveness, availability, reassurance, individual treatment, openness/informality, information, professionalism, ward organization, nurses' knowledge and ward environment***. These customer-defined values have provided the data to develop a scale to measure patients' satisfaction.

Dissatisfaction of Intubated Patients

For critically ill patients on assisted respiration caring behaviour is particularly important. A study in Israel by direct observation showed that nurses spent only a small proportion of their time talking to the patients. The interactions dealt with technical rather than emotional matters and consisted mostly of negative and discouraging comments rather than positive and supporting messages. Hospitalized intubated patients revealed a high degree of overall satisfaction with care on the one hand, and complaints of communication problems, anxiety and anger on the other. Interviews with discharged patients revealed that as many as a quarter of those who could remember their hospitalization reported feelings of anxiety, anger, distrust in the staff and difficulty in communication. These findings suggest that the staff needs improved communication skills. The judicious use of communication techniques may improve patient satisfaction, reduce anxiety and hasten recovery.

Spouse Abuse and Patient Dissatisfaction

A study examined the differences in patient satisfaction with physician care, between women who have been abused by spouses (or intimate partners) and those who have not. Abused women were much more likely than other women to report both poor communication and dissatisfaction with physicians. Over 90% of the abused women did not discuss the abuse with their physicians. Spouse abuse more than doubled respondents' odds of being dissatisfied with physician care. Therefore, spouse abuse creates barriers to patient-physician communication, and poor communication contributes to lower satisfaction with care. Careful interviewing by trained clinicians is essential to identify and address abusive situations and to prevent further damage to women's physical and mental health (Plichta, et al. 1996).

CAUSES OF PATIENT DISSATISFACTION

Diagnosis Related

- Failure to diagnose or false reassurance by the doctor
- Slow and lackadaisical approach by the doctor
- Disagreement with the diagnosis or causal explanations offered by the doctor
- No tests—deemed necessary by the patient—were advised
- Unwanted or unacceptable tests—as per the patient's opinion—were prescribed
- Tests did not help in reaching a diagnosis.

Treatment Related

- No drugs were advised
- Unwanted or unacceptable drugs were prescribed
- Adverse reactions were ignored as "trivial" by the doctor
- Expected treatment was not advised
- Treatment did not help.

Communication Related

- Rude, inattentive or "smoothing" doctor
- Confusion due to conflicting advice from the doctors
- Inadequate advice and explanations by the doctors.

DOCTORS' REACTIONS TO PATIENT DISSATISFACTION

i. Ask clinical questions—"*What exactly is wrong with you?*"
ii. Express empathy—"*I understand how it must feel to you.*"
iii. Show surprise or disbelief—"*Really! I do not think that should make you unhappy.*"
iv. Accept responsibility for dissatisfaction—"*It is my job to keep you satisfied.*"
v. Blame the patient for dissatisfaction—"*If you are unhappy, that is your problem.*"
vi. Blame other external factors for dissatisfaction—"*They made you unhappy.*"
vii. Talk about his/her own actions—"*What I have done is...*"
viii. Offer a solution—"*Let me tell you what to do.*"
ix. Refer to another person for solution—"*Just go and see this person.*"
x. Expect the problem to disappear in due course—"*Your problem will vanish before you realize.*"

AGGRESSION AND BLAMING TENDENCY

Averill's "rule model of anger" states that *people with stronger norms against aggression will account for their own angry aggression by interpreting it as passion, that is externally caused and is uncontrollable,* more than people with weaker norms against aggression. In other words, persons with a "short fuse"—one who is easily provoked—are more likely to blame themselves for their anger. A less aggressive person is more likely to label his/her anger as *a response to the external factors* (Egerton, 1988).

The rule implies that when things go wrong in healthcare, *a passive patient is more likely to blame the hospital and its personnel for the mishap.* This appears contrary to our common belief but seems to be true. A 'short-fused' person may quickly *blow his top* when things go wrong but soon cools down. It is the compliant, co-operative and *nice* patient who, when upset over an adverse outcome, is more likely to blame and sues the hospital for damages. A smart physician is the one who manages not to provoke the latter.

PROMOTING PATIENT SATISFACTION

In a recent study in Europe on patient satisfaction in primary care settings, the following 24-item patient expectations list was generated. It conveys the wide range of topics and issues that have to be addressed to promote patient satisfaction.

Patient Expectations List

I would like the doctor to:

- Understand my problem for which I came to see him/her today
- Be attentive to me
- Make it easy for me to explain my problems
- Examine me thoroughly
- Explain thoroughly about my treatment
- Explain me what the symptoms that I have mean
- Refer me to the hospital for treatment
- Explain my emotional problems
- Treat me as a person, not only a patient
- Understand my ideas about what is wrong with me
- Prescribe me some medication
- Sympathise with me for my problem
- Show a personal interest in my situation
- Talk about other matters, not related to health
- Explain the meanings of some tests that were done earlier
- Explain me how to stay healthy (diet, exercise, lifestyle, etc).

I would like to:

- Be sure nothing is wrong with me
- Know the results from some tests
- Know more about medications that I am taking, or going to take (how they work, possible side-effects)
- Know if I am likely to have any problems in future
- Know what is the likely course of my health problem
- Get help with some emotional problems
- Be referred to a specialist for treatment of my health problem
- Get some tests done to find out what is wrong with me.

SUMMARY

Professionals have to learn to 'tune in to' patient responses that indicate dissatisfaction. They need to cultivate communication habits that promote patient satisfaction.

BIBLIOGRAPHY

1. Aarflot V, et al. Do physicians know if their patients are satisfied? A study in general practice carried out by medical students. [Norwegian] 1994; 114:3579-82.
2. Ben-Ami-Lozover S. Benbassat J. [Communication with intubated patients]. [Hebrew] Harefuah. 1996;130:806-10 & 880, Jun 16 (MEDLINE abstract).
3. Delbanco TL, Stokes DM, Cleary PD, EdgmanLevitan S, Walker JD, Gerteis M, Daley J. Medical patients' assessments of their care during hospitalization: insights for internists. Journal of General Internal Medicine 1995; 10:679-85.
4. Egerton M. Passionate women and passionate men: sex differences in accounting for angry and weeping episodes. British Journal of Social Psychology 1988;27:51-66.
5. Hall JA, Irish JT, Roter DL, Ehrlich CM, Miller LH. Satisfaction, gender, and communication in medical visits. Medical Care 1994; 32:1216-31.
6. Levinson W. et al. Physician-patient communication. The relationship with malpractice claims among primary care physicians and surgeons. JAMA 1997; 277:553-9.
7. Plichta SB, Duncan MM, Plichta L, Spouse abuse, patient-physician communication, and patient satisfaction. American Journal of Preventive Medicine 1996; 12:297-303.
8. Thomas LH, MacMillan J, McColl E, Priest J, Hale C. Bond S. Obtaining patients' views of nursing care to inform the development of a patient satisfaction scale. International Journal for Quality in Health Care. 1995;7:153-63.
9. Zebiene E, Svab I, Sapoka V, Kairys J, Dotsenko M, Radic S, et al. Agreement in patient-physician communication in primary care: A study from Central and Eastern Europe. Patient Education and Counseling 2008; 73:246-50.

PRACTICAL EXERCISES

Role-play on handling the dissatisfied patients:

1. A simulated patient with chronic disease (Asthma, Migraine, Low backache etc.) dissatisfied with medical management.
2. An acute problem with uncertain outlook such as short fever- presumably viral in nature.
3. A simulated patient who has had adverse effects with many anti-hypertensive drugs.

CHAPTER

19

Negotiating Skills

> *If you wish to converse with me, define your terms.*
>
> —Voltaire

INTRODUCTION

A good outcome makes the patient overlook any dissatisfaction with healthcare services. A positive outcome may also justify the expenditure incurred and the risks and discomfort faced by the patient during the treatment. But if the outcome is adverse, the patient may complain about poor service, poor communication, high costs, unacceptable risks and question the competence of the treating professional.

It is better to prevent such dissatisfaction by being proactive and use the following steps:

- Adopt 'guidance-co-operation' model of decision-making by partnership so that the patient's preferences are incorporated in all the major treatment decisions (see Chapter 6)
- Handle risk analysis without posing to be omnipotent. The patient's trust in "scientific omnipotence" of a doctor can easily degenerate into "paranoid distrust". *Realistic optimism* is prudent.

PATIENTS' REACTION TO ADVERSE OUTCOME

- Subconsciously blame the doctor for smooth talking, for covering up and for disbelieving the patient
- If adverse outcome results in chronic incapacity, develop hostility against the doctor/s, the hospital/s, a system of medicine, or projected on to other doctors
- Fatalistic acceptance ("It is my fate," or "I brought it on myself," etc.)
- Aggravate discomfort to gain attention.

DOCTORS' REACTIONS TO ADVERSE OUTCOME

- Threat to self-image (*What will others think of me?*)
- Feelings of guilt (*What have I done?*)

- Deny that any adverse outcome has occurred (*This is not unexpected. It is OK*).
- Inability to face the hostility of the patient and his/her relatives
- Clam up due to fear of litigation
- Hint and attempt to end doctor-patient relationship.

DOs

- Do not disown the patient or the problem; arrange for its management
- Allow the patient to express his/her concerns, hopes and hostility
- Full disclosure after adverse outcome
- Give adequate time; time heals
- Review doctor-patient relationship and mutually decide to end it.

If a doctor does all this, often, to the doctor's surprise, the bonds will become stronger!

NEGOTIATING AFTER ADVERSE EVENTS

In a clinical decision, either side may inadvertently commit an error of judgement, an oversight or a misunderstanding. In the spirit of mutual 'give and take', do not hesitate to ask to negotiate. There may be an opportunity for gaining goodwill, especially if the patient's side has committed the mistake.

An example is neuro-paralytic reaction after taking Semple vaccine for rabies prophylaxis. The patient (or the relatives) may want to avoid spending money for buying a purified vaccine and agree to take the "free vaccine". However, if the patient unfortunately gets the one in thousand adverse reactions, the relatives may feel responsible and guilty and will look for ways of passing on the guilt to someone else, especially the doctor. It is better to negotiate with them before they launch into any legal action. Even though in most cases, the doctors win litigation against them, the adverse publicity does untold hardship, mental stress and damage to self-esteem.

Make the Patient/Relatives Look Good

In the preceding case, it is better to negotiate than blame the patient or the relatives for being "penny wise and pound foolish". That will only increase the guilt and increase the intensity of witch-hunting and 'blame-passing'. During negotiations, it is useful to enhance the climate. Find ways to make their key negotiators look good. You could say, "It is easy to be wise after the event; how could anyone know that this person would be the one in thousand to suffer?" Continue on similar risks we routinely accept while crossing a road or travelling in a train or by flight.

Keep Long-range Perspective in Mind

In acute adverse events, the relatives tend to be nervous, jumpy and tend to react to the immediate concerns. Stress on the long-term outlook and coax them to adopt a similar viewpoint. Time is indeed a great healer in more than one way; most patients recover from the adverse reaction and most relatives cool down and appreciate your efforts to contain the damage.

Keep the Right People Involved

Keep the right people in your own set-up or network involved in the aspects of follow-through. For example, the neuro-paralytic reaction will need a competent neurologist to examine and advice; the case may need ventilator support and intensive care. Arrange for all these.

Look for Value Enhancements

Many patients have other health problems. You may get them treated as a goodwill gesture as a part of negotiated settlement. One of my close friends, whose car hit an elderly female, used this tactic; he got her other orthopedic, dental and medical problems attended to along with the treatment of the accidental injuries. The woman and her family were thankful for the win-win gesture.

Protect Future Bargaining Strength

In the era of Consumer Protection Act (COPRA), some patients try to squeeze maximum benefits out of an adverse event. When faced with such a situation, do not reveal your trump cards for defense. Protect your bargaining power either for on-court or off-court settlement.

Summary

- Always negotiate with the patient after an adverse outcome; earlier the better
- Recognize give-and-take opportunities during a negotiation
- Renegotiate any error, oversight or misunderstanding
- Enhance a win-win climate following the negotiation
- Keep the long-range perspective in mind. Time heals
- Keep the right people in your organization involved in the follow-through
- Protect the future bargaining strength.

CULTIVATING NEGOTIATING SKILLS

When a patient threatens to go for legal redress of any adverse outcome following a procedure or treatment, we need to prepare emotionally, as well as to arm ourselves with information, prior to negotiating for an out-of-court settlement. Most litigation follows unfriendly, arrogant or hostile reactions from the doctor or his/her representatives. Face-to-face negotiation is an art and a skill. It is useful to learn it in these days of Consumer Protection Act.

Plan Adequately

Consider how far you are willing to concede. There are some obvious human errors—leaving objects within the patient or operating on the wrong person or wrong side—which cannot be explained away. Convincing the aggrieved party that it was not a malafide act, that it was a genuine human error and that you are willing to try and negotiate an acceptable solution will be a good starting point.

On the other hand, if a patient threatens to sue you for an unfortunate adverse outcome, which is part of the innate risks in the treatment process, then you should gather all the relevant information and be ready to tackle the issue face-to-face.

Be Strong in Information Gathering

Information gathering happens during both planning and face-to-face meeting. The sooner we can understand all of the patient's objectives, demands, and requests, the more usefully we can discuss the trade-off process and settle the issue.

The basic negotiating strategy is to replace concession with trade-off. The sooner we have all the relevant information, the more effectively we can do that. Information is power in hard negotiations. For example, if we can convince the patient that we have enough information to show that the adverse outcome was part of the built-in risks of the treatment and not due to negligence or malpractice, then we can negotiate from a position of strength.

Negotiate Internally First

One truism in many COPRA cases is that the patients accuse the doctors or the hospitals of making unrealistic promises. This is partly true. Some doctors are so concerned about losing a case to another doctor if they do not agree to a patient's demand, however unacceptable it might be. They readily concede to such unrealistic demands or expectations (without discussing the risk-benefit and cost-benefit issues) and hope for the best. A good example is that of a cosmetic surgeon in the USA, who agreed to perform penile enhancement on an elderly man with chronic cardiac disease, *without informing his wife* (the man wanted to surprise her). It was indeed a great shock to her when the patient died after the surgery. She sued the surgeon successfully as according to law, no doctor can harm a patient just because the patient says so.

Another common scene is when a patient claims that the doctor gave a guarantee, when at best, it was only discussed, and more often, was merely the patient's assumption. The law says it is the doctor's responsibility to clarify assumptions, to define risk, cost and benefit, and to discuss these with the patient before s/he assumes a commitment. Negotiate internally and go into all the aspects of the case, especially the case records and the consent form.

Flexible Mindset Helps

To go into a negotiation with a clear set of objectives is good. However, to go into it with a totally non-negotiable list of items is bad. It ties you up as well as the patient, generates frustration, and invites deadlock.

Put Yourself in the Patient's Shoes

We go into negotiations knowing our objectives, sensing our leverage, realizing our constraints, and concerned about the risks of a failed negotiation. Patients are thinking about the same things from their perspective. Yet, how often do we take time to view the problem from the patient's perspective?

We can guess what some of their objectives may be. But do we consider what they may view as limitations to their leverage or how they see our leverage? Do we consider what they may be worried about if talks end in a deadlock? Do we understand some of the influences in their life-world, which may affect our negotiation?

Do Not Respond too Quickly to Each Demand

This is similar to giving concessions too early, but may involve an array of secondary issues and details. Try first to get the patient's complete set of demands and requests on the table before responding. Once you understand the patient's complete list, it gives you the opportunity to tie various items together, to offer trade-offs, and, in some cases, to merely side-step unimportant items.

Call Time-outs to Cool Things Down

Some people seem to feel incompetent if they cannot respond to a patient's demand immediately. Responding inappropriately is far more incompetent than calling time-out. Find a way to call time-out, to take time to think, or to check with somebody. You can say, "I'll have to get back to you on that." Ironically, time-outs are most effective when the time pressure is on.

Do Not Give Concessions Too Early

This is partly due to poor preparation. Since we know the patient will probably ask for a concession, we should be prepared for it. Yet, repeatedly, we agree to some concession very early on in a negotiation without even testing it. Agreeing to concession demands too quickly teaches the patient bad habits. Respond to those demands with the reasons why your offer is at that level. Find out what other concessions the patient may be seeking. In addition, when you do respond to a concession demand, respond with a trade-off suggestion rather than a concession.

Do Not Let Egos Interfere

The professional to whom "winning" is more important than "striking a good deal" is dangerous. Many times we can strike a better deal if we can make the patient feel he has "won" a little more than we have.

Be Attentive in Follow-through

The important thing is to understand the difference between "follow-up" and "negotiations follow-through". Negotiations follow-through involves looking for negotiating problems and opportunities and setting the stage for future negotiations until the issue is resolved.

CHARACTERISTICS OF EFFECTIVE NEGOTIATORS

They Plan and Prepare

- They may spend days in preparing for a large and involved team negotiation or just five minutes to plan a short, routine negotiation
- They get themselves ready both cerebrally and emotionally to negotiate
- They have clearly-defined negotiating objectives.

They Negotiate Internally First

- They gain the internal commitments to fulfil any commitments made during the negotiation
- They are clear as to how much risk the management is willing to take

- They understand internal priorities, e.g. case-load versus quality, risk of adverse media exposure versus payment of "silence-money", quick settlement versus protracted legal battle, etc.

They are Creative

- They find ways to reshape the solution toward a win-win situation where both the parties gain
- They look for new trade-offs and combinations
- They are proactive and keep asking, "What if..."

They are Willing to Take Reasonable Risks

- They are willing to walk away
- They do not feel compelled to respond to every demand
- They are disciplined to courteously "hang tough".

SUMMARY

Try to develop the characteristics of an effective negotiator and sharpen your negotiating skills. It will enable you to be pro-active and prevent succumbing to unrealistic patient demands and expectations. It will also empower you to cope with adverse events whenever they occur.

BIBLIOGRAPHY

1. Applegate WB. Physician management of patients with adverse outcomes. Arch Int. Med. 1986; 146: 2249-52.
2. Negotiation follow-through by Robert Kellar; Published 2/15/99 (www.salesdoctor.com).
3. Negotiation Skills by Robert Kellar, ©1996 (www.salesdoctor.com).

PRACTICAL EXERCISES

1. Video triggers of negotiation scenes followed by Group Discussion.
2. Simulation Role-play: Students act out doctor-patient dyads after an adverse outcome.

CHAPTER

20

Patient Centered Practice

Mahatma Gandhi reminded us (the health care professionals) that the patients are the reason of our existence and the patient does us a favour by seeking our advice and service.

INTRODUCTION

"Just as the molecular and chemistry oriented sciences were adopted as the 20th century medical paradigm, incorporation of the patient's perspective into a relationship-centered medical paradigm has been suggested as appropriate for the 21st century. It is the medical dialogue that provides the fundamental vehicle through which therapeutic relationship is defined." (Roter, 2000)

Today's patients expect -

- An adequate solution, one that solves the problem as promised.
- To be partners in decision making; not just a care seeker-provider relationship.
- Valueadded service, i.e. healthcare with courtesy and comfort.

Those of us who are willing to satisfy today's more demanding, more sophisticated patient will survive and prosper. Those who refuse to change may not. The following tips may help one to make the positive changes necessary to move into the new paradigm for quality healthcare in the 21st Century.

THREE INITIAL STEPS TO PATIENT FRIENDLINESS

Learn About Patient Friendly Initiative

Patient care service is not only about doctor-patient dyad; it is everything that goes on when a patient enters a hospital. It is an attitude shared by every employee that meeting every patient's needs is paramount. Extraordinary service is having everyone in your healthcare set up sincerely care about meeting the complete needs of every single patient.

Instead of a security guard near the front door, a receptionist would receive the patients, whose job is to greet them and direct them to the department.

During the first few visits to any large hospital, most patients are confused about where to find various places. In most hospitals, if an employee was asked, "Where would we find Surgery OP?" we would expect the response to be either, "That is not my department" or "Look in second floor." Instead, in a patient friendly hospital, the employee would walk with us a few steps to show the way, or give directions until it was clear to us what we had to do.

Then there is bill payment section. Every time a patient makes a payment, the cashier would read the name off the hospital card and later says something like, "Thank you, Mr. Raju. Have a good day."

Apply Expert Knowledge to Individualize Case Management

When our patients talk about their needs and what they are looking for (in healthcare), we do not have the mental prowess to take in every little detail of their needs and expectations. We need to start with a standard case management option with which we are familiar and then look for the subtle differences that characterise each patient's unique situation.

The only way to achieve this capability is to first achieve mastery of your area of expertise. Secondly, develop skills to listen and identify the unique needs of each of your patients. Then, when an individual patient starts talking about his/her special needs, you would not have any difficulty in individualising therapy: the management plan must suit each patient; the patient must not be forcefitted into a plan. (See table on patient centeredness)

Under-promise, Over-deliver

- Never promise or raise a strong expectation for anything unless you are virtually sure that you can meet the expectation. It includes anything you do for a patient, e.g. giving information or attending to a patient on time.
- Always promise your patients a little less care than you are capable of delivering.
- Always deliver a little more care than you promise your patients.

Behaviors of a patient-centered physician and an empowered patient

Patient-centered professional	*Empowered patient*
Complete acceptance of patients as human beings with health problems.	Feels tranquil, confident and secure during the consultation.
Realises the need of every patient to be informed. If a patient does not know what is happening, she/he can not collaborate, or take responsibility for her/his health.	The patient tries to understand and to take responsibility for one's own health. Co-operates with the care provider in shared decision making.
Feels and acts like a person; not an authority figure. Discourages dependence and encourages self- determination by the patients.	Feels validated as a person because of the adult-adult relationship. Does not behave as a dependent patient looking up to a doctor.
Listens, observes, questions and learns what is necessary to know about patients, their values, history and environment in order to gather a total picture of illness.	Expresses in depth, without holding back information that could be important; is not afraid to disclose personal details, nor worried about how s/he might be judged. Takes responsibility for adhering to therapy.
Explains important side effects, the benefits and risks of treatments and surgery.	Decides after being informed and accepts the corresponding risks. For complex decisions, seeks counsel from the professional.
Does not impose own opinion about sensitive issues like birth control or about the use of new medications or surgery.	Has the right to change opinions, to make mistakes and learn from them.

Contd...

Contd...

Is flexible, understanding and uncomplicated- "a person just like me" Shows an emotion like empathy, affection or admiration (as opposed to seduction, which is an abuse of his/her position and the patient's psychologically fragile state). Listens and pays attention to the patient's fears, intuition and feelings.Takes pride in being a professional who is consulted because of his/her expertise in the field.	Does not become infatuated with the doctor; is clear about the professional's intentions and attends appointments enthusiastically. Knows that s/he is understood, and is thus able to acknowledge her own worth and feel secure. Looks for professional help that s/he values and feels is necessary to get better.

TIPS FOR PATIENT CENTERED PRACTICE

Problemsolving Solutions

Specialization and high-tech medicine has rendered healthcare more complex and challenging than ever before. Patients want not just services but solutions to their problems. Your ability to analyze your patients' problems and solve those problems at a reasonable cost will create high-perceived value and continuing demand for your expertise. (Computer professionals have realized it long ago and now they offer not merely *services* but *solutions.*) It is high time we also adopted such outcome-oriented problem solving approach to healthcare.

Realistic Guarantee

Many patients harbour a fear that the care they get may not meet their expectations or that any improvement in health may not last long. Of course, "There are no guarantees in Medicine" but when you put a guarantee on *the quality of your service*, you provide peace of mind. Just make sure you back up your words; also ensure that your patient understands that *you vouch for the quality and not the outcome of the healthcare process.* When patients tells you, "Doctor, even if I die, it does not matter; I want to be treated here/by you", then you know that realistic guarantee has been understood by them.

Perceived Quality

Everything you do that enhances the patients' perception of quality service creates more value in their mind.

Follow-up Support

Patients using hightech products (insulin-pen, pacemaker, home nebuliser therapy, Holter monitoring, etc.) need adequate training to use them properly. Any training that enables your patient to feel competent in handling them, adds value to the healthcare. Such patients pleasantly surprised by the level of service you provide will be your best advertisers. Conduct patientsatisfaction surveys to determine their perceptions about your service. Measure the difference between what you promise and what you really deliver.

Save Patients' Time and Money

The old cliché, "Time is money" certainly applies to your patients as much as it applies to you. Most professionals ignore this aspect totally. When you offer advice that saves your patient's time, money or effort, you would be viewed as a truly professional consultant. A few moments of your time, along with your technical expertise, adds immeasurable value to the services you provide.

Advance Notice of Changes

Everyone likes to get useful information. By providing your patients with useful insights into what is new in Medicine that is of relevance to them, you add value to your service. Keep them aware of changes that will affect them, both positively and negatively; an example would be to inform your diabetic patients about newer treatment options. Such information adds value to your service and your relationship.

Personalized Attention

Everyone likes to feel special. Healthcare today, especially with multispeciality 'piecemeal' care becoming the norm, leaves most patients without personal acknowledgement from care providers. When you make a practice of paying special attention to your patients, you give them something most other doctors fail to deliver. Appointment reminder cards or anniversary cards (acknowledging each year of your relationship) add real value to any relationship.

Consider patient as a person who has a name, hopes, life-goals, priorities and expectations. Many hospitals treat patients as "non-persons" who do not count except as a case to be treated; the feelings, privacy needs and priorities of non-persons do not matter; one can perform intrusive questioning and physical examination on them. This should stop if you want them to feel that they get personal attention.

Unexpected Addons

As a health professional, who provides quality service, your job is to meet and exceed our patients' expectations. Look for ways by which you can go beyond the commitment you make when you accept a patient for care. Throw in something that costs little to you but adds convenience (ambulance pickup and dropback), or educational value (patient information brochures) to your service. Make it a point to deliver more than what patients expect. That is what "Quality" is all about - *exceeding patient expectation.*

Special Packaging of Documents and Reports

You can spruce up the perceived value of your service by simply putting it into a better-looking package. Creative packaging that adds convenience, attractiveness, functionality or longer life to hospital documents and reports makes it a better value for your customers. Excellent packaging of scan-images, X-ray films and colour coded lab reports are some examples.

Help Form Support/Self-help Groups

Thanks to the Internet, there are support and self-help groups for almost all health problems access to any of them is easy. Encourage and guide your patients with chronic diseases to join an appropriate group. Web-sites and Usenet groups are available for almost all the chronic illnesses.

Help in Payment Assistance

Payment of healthcare expenses is a major concern for all except those who are well insured or wealthy. You can organise some assistance to the needy through deferred payment, easy loans, donor aid etc.

PREVENTING PATIENT DROP-OUT

Today, the patients are often so disappointed with the kind of healthcare they receive that they go elsewhere. The doctor/hospital is noticed, gets the patient, and then because of bad manners, rudeness, indifference, poor follow up, bad service, slow response etc, loses the patient and also a bit of the reputation. It is not difficult to get patients to consult once. It is much more difficult to retain them so that they return to you whenever they have health problems.

Common Reasons for Losing Patients to Follow-up

Today, patients, especially the urban lot, have plenty of options in seeking healthcare. The common reasons why a professional or a hospital loses patients are:

- Not listening to the patient; telling the solution before hearing the problems fully.
- Putting money or profits ahead of service.
- Complacency brought about by success. Therefore, not paying attention to the patients or the competition; isolationism or "head in the sand" attitude to obvious lapses.
- Lack of the spirit of teamwork (personnel blaming each other or whining "it's not my job.")
- Not valuing patients' time.
- Lip service, smoothing or worse, lying.
- Lack of proper training, recognition, or retention of personnel.

Re-orienting Healthcare to Patient Satisfaction

Effective patient care requires consistent behavior from every employee whom patients encounter. To re-orient the mindset of healthcare personnel to "Patient-centered service", start with these Ten Commandments.

Be Interested

Do not act as if you are fed up with your profession and hate seeing patients. People like consulting professionals who are happy to be in their profession. Patients would prefer to spend more time and money to get healthcare that is friendly, accommodating and interested in them. Some of the ways to show you care are - having up-to-date knowledge and skills, and knowing who does what in your set up, so that you can efficiently guide the patients to find someone concerned with solving their problems.

The Patient Deserves Your Best at all Times

The essence of professionalism is to do one's best regardless of the time of day, personal problems or prevailing mood. If you have worked late last night, it should not become your patient's problem. The patient also deserves your best, regardless of your training, length of service, or any other prevailing professional attitude.

You may be only days away from finishing residency, just married, or waiting to ride your new car. You may be whining that the unit chief just does not understand. It may be your first week on the job. If you permit these and hundred other situations like them to become problems to your patients, then they will seek out some other healthcare set up. When you can not do the best for a case, call for help or refer to a better set up.

Shift the Responsibility only when Needed

Whoever hears a problem owns the problem. How often have you been transferred on the telephone several times before you finally got to the right person? Do not get upset when patients bring up a complaint that does not pertain to your speciality. Acknowledge the problem, explain its basis and help them solve it; refer the case when indicated - not just to "get the patient of my back."

Do not be too Busy for Your Patients

Do not make it difficult for them to consult you. How many times have you felt that you are an interruption in an employee's day or workload? Have you ever been made to feel that you should have no problem with a service and any fault is because of your own mistakes?

The Patient is not Always Right

However, the goal is not to discredit, embarrass, belittle or challenge patients in a destructive way. What we need to do is discover the source or cause of their incorrect perceptions, beliefs or attitudes. The next step is to determine if the hospital has contributed in some way to these incorrect feelings or if their source is some other hospital, the media, or their friends and relatives.

The Patient is Never Totally Wrong

There is always some element of a patient's perception that is a true reflection of reality as they see it. The patient can be a teacher for us if we will keep an open mind and receptive, neutral demeanour. A patient can give a feedback to us on our communication skill, management methods etc.

If You Must use Technology, Make it User-Friendly

Due to computer crashes, a patient has five cancellations of a minor surgery. When he rings up to speak with a responsible doctor, he has to spend a lot of valuable time -'on hold'- listening to endless music. Never inflict user-unfriendly technology on your patients. They will drop out at the earliest.

Say What You Will Do, and Do What You Say

Follow through, keep your promises, honour your commitments and keep patients informed of your progress. Patients will tend to be more understanding, patient and tolerant if you communicate with them with integrity and in a timely manner.

Keep Private Things Private

Patients are not interested in your personal problems or hospital politics. Patients do not have the time to hear, nor are they interested in hearing, about who did what to whom and why in your hospital. They do not want to know you are looking for another job. Sharing private, confidential or personal information, is in poor taste and unprofessional. It also makes patients wonder how much of their secrets will remain so with you.

Be Proactive

Think ahead of the patient with a problem-solving attitude. To survive and prosper in the new century, it will require hospitals and all their employees to think well ahead of their patients' potential future desires, problems and needs. If you wait for patients to bring their problems to you or to communicate their future desires or needs with you, it may be too late.

SUMMARY

Every patient's expectation for healthcare is unique and deserves your flexibility, attention and an extra effort to meet and exceed their expectations. That is what quality service is all about. Great healthcare service is a never ending pursuit of excellence to keep the patients so satisfied that they tell others of the way they were treated in your place. If they do, you would be among the top 5% of healthcare facilities. The other 95% fall short of that mark.

BIBLIOGRAPHY

1. Articles on Quality of Service and Client centredness in www.mindtools.com.
2. Gremigni P, Sommaruga M, Peltenburg M. Validation of the Health Care Communication Questionnaire (HCCQ) to measure outpatients' experience of communication with hospital staff. Patient Education and Counseling 2008;71:57–64.
3. Links on 'Patient-centredness' in www.bmj.com and www.medscape.com.
4. Roter D. The enduring and evolving nature of the patient–physician relationship. Patient Education and Counseling 2000;39:5–15.
5. Roter Interaction Analysis System (RIAS). URL: http://riasworks.com/resources.html (accessed on 09-09-2010; *vide* Annexure-4)
6. Smith RC, Marshall-Dorsey AA, Osborn GG, Shebroe V, Lyles JS, Stoffelmayr BE, Van Egeren LF, Mettler J, Maduschke K, Stanley JM, Gardiner JC. Evidence-based guidelines for teaching patient-centered interviewing. Patient Education and Counseling 2000;39:27–36.
7. WHO publications on Quality of Healthcare.

PRACTICAL EXERCISES

Sample Survey and Group Discussion

Students, in small batches, can go to different wards of the hospital and conduct a sample survey of patient expectation and perceived shortfall in service, using the following checklist (Gremigni, et al. 2008).

Domain-1. Problem solving
Clear requests
Clear information
Solve the patient problem
Manage the difficulties
Keep calm

Domain-2. Respect
Respect of patients' needs
Courtesy
Consideration of patients' privacy

Domain-3. Lack of hostility
Polite requests (versus Aggressive requests)
Polite answers (versus Aggressive answers)
Relaxed approach (versus Rushed approach)

Domain-4. Non verbal immediacy
Eye contact
Visible Smile

Then they conduct a group discussion to identify common expectations, commonly perceived shortfalls and possible ways of meeting their expectations. The tutor can highlight the two major components in perceived quality viz., *Scientific Medicine* - domain-1 of the checklist and *Art of Medicine* - the emotional and behavioural aspects of healthcare - domains 2,3,&4 of the checklist.

A more detailed and specific feedback can be given, using RIAS rating scale (*vide* Annexure-4) instead of the above checklist.

Simulation Role-play

Basic Patient-centered Interviewing:

Use the checklist given below to rate the steps taken for patient centered interview and give feedback.

Basic patient-centered interviewing method (Smith, 2000)

i. Setting the stage for the interview (Step 1)
   a. Welcome the patient
   b. Use the patient's name
   c. Introduce self and identify specific role
   d. Ensure patient readiness and privacy

e. Remove barriers to communication
f. Ensure comfort and put the patient at ease

ii. Chief complaint/agenda setting (Step 2)
a. Indicate time available
b. Indicate own needs; e.g., take history and perform physical examination
c. Obtain list of all issues patient wants to discuss; e.g., specific symptoms, requests, expectations, understanding
d. Summarize and finalize the agenda; negotiate specifics if too many agenda items

iii. Nonfocused interviewing (Step 3)
a. Open-ended beginning question
b. 'Nonfocusing' open-ended skills: silence, neutral utterances, nonverbal encouragement
c. 'Focusing' open-ended inquiry also appropriate if needed to get patient talking: echoing, summary, requests
d. Closed-ended questions for clarification
e. Obtain additional data from the following sources: nonverbal cues, physical characteristics, autonomic changes, accouterments, and environment

iv. Focused interviewing (Step 4)
a. Obtain personal description of the physical symptoms [Focusing open-ended skills]
b. Extend the story to the broader, personal context of the symptoms [Focusing open-ended skills]
c. Develop an emotional focus [Emotion-seeking skills]
d. Address the emotion(s) [Emotion-handling skills]
e. Use the cycle of 'core dynamic skills' repeatedly (focused open-ended skills, emotion-seeking skills, emotion-handling skills) to better identify and deepen the story
f. Conclude and address other current issues

v. Transition to the doctor-centered process (Step 5)
a. Brief summary
b. Check accuracy
c. Indicate that both content and style of inquiry will change if the patient is ready.

Adjusting Interview Techniques to Match the Type of Patient-Doctor Dyad

Four dyads can be simulated:

i. Paternalistic doctor & Passive patient
ii. Paternalistic doctor & Empowered patient
iii. Patient centered doctor & Passive patient
iv. Patient centered doctor & Empowered patient

In the debriefing plenary session, the importance of matching a doctor's role to that of the patient's passivity or empowerment has to be highlighted. Dyads 2 and 3 show mismatch and the resultant dissatisfaction. Dyad 1 and 4 are matched and both are good examples of patient-centeredness, which result in satisfaction.

CHAPTER

21

Prudent Practice

> *Only one who devotes himself to a cause with his whole strength and soul can be a true master. For this reason, mastery demands All of a person.*
>
> \- Albert Einstein

The task of the physician is two-fold: to understand the patient and to understand the disease. There is a well tried clinical method for understanding diseases, but no equivalent method for understanding patients. However, even medical tasks are not always as scientifically proven as we would like to believe: there is much inter-observer variation, which affects the accuracy and variability of assumed clinical facts—i.e., when reading of mammographic images. Furthermore, diagnosis of a disease is affected by a doctor's personal experiences, and is not always just a matter of objectively observable facts (Malterud 2001).

Being prudent is half way to being wise. The ultimate aim of improved doctor-patient dyad is to help solve patients' problems prudently (and wisely). Prudent practice improves patient outcome and patient satisfaction, while reducing the risk of litigation. Prudent practice needs mindfulness and a sustained and multi-pronged effort to improve oneself as a skilled professional.

LEVELS OF MINDFULNESS

Mindfulness, which is essential to practice prudently, may be classified in an ascending order thus:

1. Denial or externalisation. (No attention to case details) - "Spinal level prescribing" is a good example.
2. Imitation - adopt a role model. (Try and behave like the senior doctor)
3. Curiosity to understand ideas, facts and concepts. (Reflect on the main messages in each case)
4. Curiosity to understand emotions and attitudes. (Reflect on the patient's feelings and personality)
5. Insight - holistic perspective of the patients' problem. (View a problem in all its dimension)

6. Presence, generalisation and incorporation into future practice. (Consider the learning points in the current case that may be of use in future practice)

One must try to be at the highest attainable level of mindfulness during clinical dyads. For novices, this may prove difficult in crowded out patient settings but is possible while examining in-patients.

TEN CHARACTERISTICS OF PRUDENT PRACTICE

1. Presence - totally attentive presence in mind, body and spirit.
2. Active observation of the problem, the patient and oneself.
3. Peripheral vision and peripheral listening to pick up cues and leads.
4. Pre-attentive processing (explained below).
5. Critical curiosity and adoption of the mindset of a novice.
6. Open mind to see the clinical practice as it is, and not as you want it to be.
7. Willingness to examine and weed out prejudice and generalisation.
8. Awareness of areas of incompetence and the humility to accept them.
9. Compassion and empathy based on insight.
10. Facilitate the patient to perceive his/her illness in a holistic way.

CULTIVATING MINDFULNESS

While attending to a patient, our awareness level is of two types:

- *Explicit awareness* which is formally learnt in medical schools.
- *Tacit awareness,* which refers to intuitive knowledge about patient's background and quick recognition of the syndrome even before explicit awareness confirms it.

Pre-attentive processing is another term that refers to the ability of experienced professionals to recognise a syndrome tacitly, quickly and almost subconsciously.

Tacit and explicit awareness could relate to four types of knowledge used in clinical practice:

i. *Prepositional knowledge* consisting of facts, concepts, theories and principles acquired from learning resources and from instructors.

ii. *Personal knowledge* consists of facts, insight, intuition and interpretation that help in clinical practice.

iii. *Experts' knowledge* takes into account finer details like clinical context, cost factor, convenience, the values and preferences of patients etc. It is impossible to make explicit all aspects of professional competence. As practitioners, we apply a broad range of experiential knowledge and strategies that are hardly mentioned in the textbooks. This tacit and practical knowing inherent in clinical practice is often referred to as the art of medicine (Malterud 2001).

iv. *Process knowledge,* i.e., knowing ways of accomplishing a task or solving a problem. "Know-how" refers to the ability to apply the above (knowledge) to get things done (action); in addition to knowledge and intelligence, emotional quotient plays a big part in this.

Real Life Examples

1. If an undiagnosed outpatient with 'general weakness' casually remarked, "I can eat *Idli* but not *Chappatti,"* most of us would just nod and carry on with 'case disposal.' However,

a '*mindful*' resident picked up the clue (by pre-attentive processing), worked up the case and proved it as myasthenic syndrome (see chapter-3).

2. A female patient in her forties presented in 1975 with pyrexia of unknown origin (PUO) for 3 weeks. She had been giving bedside care for her sick daughter for over 6 months. Her daughter had recently died after PUO of about 6 months despite treatment with anti-malarial, antibiotics and anti TB therapy. They lived in Madras and had never travelled outside the city for three years previously. The treating resident initially diagnosed it as a case of acute Leishmaniasis, which amused the seniors.
   Non-response of the daughter to empirical therapy for all the common causes of PUO, her demise in 6 months and her mother getting the same type of illness after staying at her bedside for several weeks were the reasons for the diagnosis. All tests were initially negative but were positive for Leishmaniasis when repeated after three more weeks. It also happened the first such case reported in the hospital. She responded well to treatment.
3. A female patient, apparently in her middle age, was brought with pallor and hypotension following a few bouts of mild diarrhoea. Her only child was 8 years old and her age had been recorded as 26. The duty consultant observed that since the diarrhoea was not severe enough to cause hypotension or pallor, she must be a case of Sheehan's syndrome. The residents were surprised by the 'snap diagnosis' but when they elicited her history in detail, she turned out to have classical features of post-partum hypopituitarism (Sheehan's syndrome).

The consultant had shown *pre-attentive processing* in syndrome recognition and *mindfulness* in recognising paradoxes (her apparent age versus real age; her mild diarrhoea versus hypotension; pallor versus no loss of blood and no nail signs of iron deficiency).

Caution

Do not get carried away and adopt "snap diagnosis" as the way of prudent practice. The above examples highlight how mindful case examination could enable proper diagnosis to be reached. Initial impressions have to be backed up by clinical and laboratory evidences.

SECTION 3

SUMMARY

Mindful practice needs mental concentration and full attentiveness to patient details. It has to be cultivated. It helps to couple your knowledge and skills with the patient's problem ('problem-knowledge coupler'). It enables you to metamorphose from being a mere 'prescriber' to a 'problem solver'.

BIBLIOGRAPHY

1. Epstein RM. Mindful practice. JAMA. 1999; 282:833-9
2. Malterud K. The art and science of clinical knowledge: evidence beyond measures and numbers. Lancet. 2001; 358: 397-400.
3. Problem-Knowledge Coupler articles at http://www.pkc.com/articles.aspx (accessed on 19-09-2010)

PRACTICAL EXERCISES

"Six Clues" Quiz

Select diseases and syndromes relevant and appropriate to the student group. Write down diagnostic clues from history and examination findings. (Real life cases will be stranger, tougher than simulated cases). Conduct a quiz in which the case details are read out one by one. Who ever correctly tells the diagnosis first gets points. Have some penalty points for mistakes made so that mindless guesswork is not encouraged.

Students may be asked to study relevant chapters and then attend the quiz. Then mindfulness will be more meaningful and the diagnosis more scientifically arrived at.

CHAPTER

22 Telecommunication in Healthcare

The object of all work is production or accomplishment and to either of these ends, there must be forethought, system, planning, intelligence, and honest purpose, as well as perspiration. Seeming to do is not doing.

- Thomas Alva Edison

INTRODUCTION

The healthcare system suffers from enormous inefficiency because of poor communication. A retrospective Australian survey of hospital admissions found that communication problems were the most common cause of preventable disability or death, and were nearly twice as common as those due to inadequate medical skill. Despite this evidence, there has been little examination of the communication systems within health care.

Documentation in healthcare delivery systems, and communication between the health professionals in those delivery systems, is chaotic. Doctors need more training on effective use of information technology, structured data collection, and adoption of new mobile and point-of-care technologies.

PHONE ETIQUETTE

Good telephone skills are essential these days. Yet strangely, as we rely on the phone more and more, the communication skills of many people in the workforce seem to be getting worse. We all have memories of rude operators or ill-informed persons providing nothing but frustration when all we wanted was a simple answer to an uncomplicated question. Do not let this happen to your own patients or colleagues when they talk to you.

Basics of Telephone Etiquette

i. Answer the telephone (by the second or third ring!) with a warm, clear, articulate greeting that includes your name.
ii. Speak slowly and clearly. There is no substitute for clarity.

iii. Smile, you are on the telephone. People can hear the extra warmth in your voice, even when they can not see you. By physically smiling, you will automatically appear friendlier to the ear.
iv. Know what you are talking about. You (and your employees) should be knowledgeable enough to converse about your patient's problem over the telephone without having to speculate or follow a routine dialogue.
v. In case you do not know what the other person is talking about, pleasantly and promptly refer them to someone who may do.
vi. If you must put people on hold, inform them first. Let them know if they are in for a long wait.
vii. Make sure your staff is trained to express politeness, friendliness, and helpfulness over the telephone. Just because your patients can not see you, does not mean they are not forming a clear impression of you.

NEWER MODES: SYNCHRONOUS VERSUS ASYNCHRONOUS MODE

A study by Coiera and Tombs confirms that face to face, telephone, or pager-based communication is common in hospitals and these are driven by events. Hospital communications are inefficient and commonly interrupt tasks, including patient consultations.

Interruption is related to the type of communication method chosen. Synchronous communication occurs when two individuals participate in a conversation at the same time, such as using the telephone. Asynchronous communication occurs when the exchange does not require both to be active participants at the same time, such as exchanging letters. It is a characteristic of synchronous communication that a request to speak creates an interruption, but with an asynchronous message the receiver chooses the moment to check or reply to the message.

We should use and evaluate asynchronous methods of communication, such as electronic mail or message boards, which are potentially less disruptive to professionals' work and patients' welfare.

PROBLEMS AND ATTITUDES

Time is what we want most, but what alas! We use worst.

- William Penn

Regardless of the medium used, unless there is a commitment on the part of the professional to communicate well and efficiently, inter professional communication will continue to be inefficient and error prone. A well-written referral-note may be many folds better than a hasty or purposeless teleconference. Some of the common attitudinal and procedural problems are-

- There are well known psychological costs associated with interruption, leading to diversion of attention, forgetfulness, and errors.
- The medical staff do not perceive the effect of a telephone call or a page would have on the recipient's activity. The motive is selfish in that they value completion of their own tasks over their colleagues' tasks.
- Many staff are unsure about who could assist them with a task and end up making many unsuccessful calls disturbing the work schedule of many others.

- Some of the doctors assess the urgency of a call by the number of times they were called and the origin of the call; they do not reply unless paged twice in succession, which indicates urgency.
- Similarly, failure to get a reply to a page within a short period is often taken to mean that no answer is coming.
- Problems with co-operative tasks occur when team members were geographically separated. For example, an intern and senior house officer who are physically separated can duplicate an order for an urgent ECG because they are unaware of each other's actions.
- Two senior consultants may try to communicate, involving at least two intermediaries. By the time the second consultant receives the message, it may be distorted and even cause avoidable errors.
- There seems to be a need for every one to consider carefully the effects of one's communication behaviour on one's own efficiency and effectiveness as well as on that of others.
- Professionals are highly mobile during their working day. The difficulty contacting these "moving targets" may be reduced by the use of wireless technology (such as cellular telephones.
- Early attempts to introduce message boards in order to reduce paging traffic have failed. Nursing staff did not have any feedback about when messages were likely to be read or acted on.

Some Solutions

- Provision of messaging facilities such as "group-sms", voicemail, email and social networking links such as "twitter" might succeed, partly because they can be accessed wherever staff are working. Such messaging services may need to provide acknowledgement to reassure staff that messages have been acted on.
- Many of the hospital communications are to occupants of specific roles -say, the duty doctor- rather than named individuals -say Dr Kumar. A role-based database could dynamically associate roles with names and could reduce the effort and error in seeking the personnel.
- Recipients of calls usually have no information to prioritise the calls meaningfully. If information such as the caller's identity, perceived urgency of task and nature of task can be attached to email and voicemail, it may be possible to prioritise meaningfully.
- Supporting collaboration among geographically separated team members to communicate the state of individual tasks may reduce duplication of effort and communication costs. For example, mobile computers could allow teams to work from a common task list.

SUMMARY

There are several ways in which communications between primary and secondary care may be improved. Present economic, technical, and political trends make expansion of its role imminent. Digital standards of the telecom, Internet and TV industry are achieving conformity. The cost of basic videoconferencing technology is falling. Such technology is already being used in Andhra Pradesh.

Regardless of the medium in use, the system should adopt a two-way channel with feedback loop to reduce errors and make it fool proof.

BIBLIOGRAPHY

1. "14,000 preventable deaths in Australian hospitals." BMJ 1995;310:1487.
2. Coiera EW, Tombs V. Communication behaviours in a hospital setting: an observational study. BMJ 1998; 316: 673-676.
3. Coiera EW. Medical informatics. BMJ 1995; 310: 1381-1387
4. Editorials: Communication among health professionals. BMJ 1998; 316:642.
5. Gosbee Enrico Coiera, Vanessa Tombs. Communication behaviours in a hospital setting: an observational study. BMJ 1998; 316:673-676.
6. Harrison R. Clayton W. Wallace P. Can telemedicine be used to improve communication between primary and secondary care? BMJ. 1996; 313(7069):1377-80 (discussion 1380-1).
7. Little AD. Telecommunications: can it help solve America's health care problems? Cambridge, MA: Arthur D Little, 1992.
8. "Phone Etiquette" article available at www.mindtools.com
9. Robert Harrison, William Clayton and Paul Wallace. Can telemedicine be used to improve communication between primary and secondary care? BMJ 1996;313:1377-80.

PRACTICAL EXERCISES

Simulated Phone Calls

Students can learn telephone etiquette by speaking to each other. Feedback can be given to improve their performance.

ANNEXURE

1 Transactional Analysis —Understanding of Human Interaction

I contradict myself. I contain multitudes.

—Walt Whitman.

INTRODUCTION

Eric Berne, the pioneer of Transactional Analysis (TA) said that all human interactions consist of transactions. Any transaction has two parts: a stimulus and a response. Individual transactions are usually part of a larger set. Some of these transactional sets or sequences can be direct, productive and healthy or they can be devious, wasteful and unhealthy. By analyzing and understanding transactions, it is possible for us to improve our interpersonal communication skills.

EGO STATES IN TRANSACTIONS

When people interact, they do so in one of three different ego states. An ego state is a specific way of thinking, feeling and behaving. People can behave from their *parent, child* or *adult* ego state. Studies have shown that each ego state originates from specific regions of the brain.

At any given time, our actions come from one of these three ego states. In order to be a well-functioning human being, all the three ego states must be available when needed. In some persons, one ego state may dominate to the exclusion of the other two. This is a great disadvantage and may result in maladaptation.

The Child Ego State

The ego states are fully experienced states of being, not just roles. When we are in the Child ego state we act like the child we once were. We are not putting on an act; we think, feel, see, hear and react as a three, five or eight-year-old child. The Child has all the feelings; fear, love, anger, joy, sadness, shame, etc.

- When the Child is hateful or loving, impulsive, spontaneous or playful, it is called the *Natural Child.*

- When it is thoughtful, creative or imaginative, it is called the *Little Professor.*
- When it is fearful, guilty or ashamed it is called the *Adapted Child*; the opposite is the *rebel.*

The Child is often blamed for being the source of problems because it is self-centerd, emotional, powerful and resists the suppression that comes with growing up. The Child can be seen as the source of *creativity, recreation and procreation.* It is the only source of renewal in life. When faced with a problem, the Child will create novel solutions based on intuition but these solutions may not be as reliable or feasible as the fact-based Adult decisions.

The Child ego state can be observed in children for extended periods. It is seen in grownups in situations where they have permission to let the Child out, e.g. when they hear good news, in a labor room, after a successful surgery, etc. The Child also appears for short periods in other situations, such as serious clinical discussions when it may not be desirable. In its most undesirable form it completely dominates a person's life, e.g. *addicted Child* that drives a chain smoker or an alcoholic to virtual self-destruction. The Child may also dominate for long periods in the form of depression or grief in persons who have incurred a great loss.

The Parent Ego State

The Parent ego state is like a programed robot. It is a collection of prerecorded, prejudged, prejudiced codes for living imprinted in a person during formative years. A person in the Parent ego state thinks, feels and behaves like one of his/her parents or a parental figure who influenced the person during the formative years. Therefore, the Parent is usually a generation (twenty-five years) behind the times.

The Parent arbitrarily decides, based on prejudice or assumptions, what is good or bad, and how people should live. The Parent uses old "rules" to solve problems. This is useful when there is no information or no time to use the Adult to think and decide rationally. *Voices in the Head* arise from the Parent ego state consisting of prejudged, prejudiced, preprogramed statements. These statements can be activated while we are in our Adult or Child and then we can actually hear them as "voices in our heads."

The Parent judges for or against and can be controlling or supportive.

- When the Parent is controlling and critical, the ego state is called the *Critical Parent.*
- When it is supportive, the ego state is called the *Nurturing Parent.*

The Adult Ego State

The Adult ego state of a person functions as an analytical robot. The Adult ego state uses logical thinking to solve problems making sure that child or parent do not contaminate the process. It means that to be rational and logical, we need to separate ourselves from our emotions. Nevertheless, to be rational and logical may not be the best option at all times. Pure Adult ego state has "deadening effect" on people. A professional, who uses only the Adult to relate to patients, misses a total and highly satisfying doctor-patient relationship that spans all the three ego states **(Box A1.1)**.

Being a mature human being does not mean that one should permanently be in the Adult ego state. Well-adjusted grown ups use their Parent for values, Child for emotions and Adult to control the intellect.

Box A1.1: Characteristics of true adulthood

- Accepts the responsibility of own acts without trying to alibi
- Does not indulge in self-pity; perceives and accepts the laws of compensation of nature.
- Is open-minded enough to listen thoughtfully to the opinions of others
- Accepts advice and criticism gratefully and is honestly glad for an opportunity for self-improvement
- Has outgrown the 'black and white' view of Life; realises that no person or situation is wholly good or wholly bad; is not a chronic faultfinder
- Plans things in advance rather than leaving it to the last minute
- Meets emergencies with poise
- Realizes that one is not the arbiter of the universe and that one must often adjust to other people and their convenience
- Controls temper; tolerates reasonable delays
- Is a good loser; can endure defeat and disappointment without whining or complaining
- Feelings are not easily hurt
- Does not expect special consideration from anyone
- Does not worry unduly about things he cannot help
- Does not boast or show-off in socially unacceptable ways
- Has outgrown envy and jealousy; is honestly glad when others enjoy success or good fortune.

Sometimes the Adult uses biased information from the Child or the Parent. This is known as *contamination*. Many "defense mechanisms" of the patients elicited during counseling are examples of contamination. When a contamination comes from the Parent, it is called a *prejudice*. For instance, when a patient assumes that *men are better surgeons than women are,* this message comes to the Adult from the Parent; it is a contamination because Adult accepts it as a fact without checking it against reality.

Uncritical acceptance can similarly occur with information fed by the Child in which case it is called *delusion*. A delusion is usually based on a Child's fear or hope and is accepted as reality by the Adult. For example, most advertizing gimmicks aim at 'contaminating' the Adult through the Child. An extremely important process in transactional analysis is decontamination of the Adult. This is clinically useful in counseling of unhealthy lifestyle, addictions and other self-destructive behaviors.

TRANSACTIONS—COMPLEMENTARY, CROSSED AND COVERT

Transactions occur when any person relates to any other person. Each transaction is made up a stimulus and a response and transactions can proceed from the Parent, Adult or Child of one person to the Parent, Adult or Child of another person.

Complementary and Crossed Transactions

A complementary transaction involves one ego state in each person. An example: When your Adult asks the patient's Adult, "What is your problem?" the reply is also from his/her Adult to your Adult, such as, "I have severe headache." (A with A) Communication can continue between two people as long as transactions are complementary e.g. (P with P) (C with C) (C with A) (C with P) or (P with A) **(Table A1.1).**

Table A1.1: Three types of transactions between ego states of a doctor and a patient

Complementary type	*Crossed type*	*Discount type*
Doctor (Adult) to Patient (Adult):	Doctor (Adult) to Patient (Adult):	Patient (Adult) to Doctor (Adult):
"What is your problem?"	"What is your problem?	I have severe headache."
Patient (Adult) to Doctor (Adult):	"Patient (Child) to Doctor (Parent):	"Doctor (Parent) to Patient (Child):
"I have severe headache."	- (Non-verbal Coy posturing)	"You always imagine problems!"

In a crossed transaction, the transactional response is addressed to an ego state different from the one, which started the stimulus. An example: You ask the same question to elicit the patient's problem (A to A) but the patient responds by being coy (Child to Parent). If such a response engages your nurturing parent, you may encourage and coax the patient. If it engages your critical parent, you may say some harsh words. (A to P; C to A) (C to C; P to C) are other examples of crossed transactions. Crossed transactions are important because they disrupt communication. The rule is: "*Whenever a disruption of communication occurs, a crossed transaction caused it.*"

One very important kind of crossed transaction initiated by doctors is the *discount transaction*. Here the doctor, in his/her response, completely disregards the contents of a transactional stimulus from the patient. An example: Patient—"Doctor, I was worrying about my aches and..." Doctor—"You always worry about things and make a mountain out of a mole-hill." Discounts are not always so obvious during a dyad but they are always disruptive to the patient receiving them and if repeated often, can severely disturb the patient.

Covert Transactions

Covert transactions occur when people say one thing and mean another. Covert transactions are deceptive and form the basis of "games." They have an overt (social) and a covert (psychological) level. The covert level will provide more information than the overt level in predicting what people are going to do. An important reason, a person may say one thing and mean another is that his/her Adult may be ashamed of the Child's or Parent's desires and feelings. Nevertheless, she/he acts on these desires and expresses those feelings while she/he pretends to be doing otherwise.

For instance, a diabetic patient who has a "sweet tooth" may be ashamed to acknowledge it and therefore be deceptive. He may say, "I want to totally give up eating sugar but my friends do not permit it" (Overt: Adult to Adult message, "I want to give up." Covert: Child to Parent message, "I can not give it up but blame my friends. They make me eat sugar.").

Some doctors also transact covertly, when the apparent reason told to the patient (say, for a surgical procedure) is only cover a covert reason (say, desire to operate or to make more money).

STROKES

Stroking is the recognition that one person gives to another during transactions. Strokes are essential to a person's life. Without them, Berne said, the 'spinal cord will shrivel up'.

It has been shown that a very young child needs actual physical strokes or they may suffer from "sensory deprivation". Adults need fewer physical strokes. They learn to exchange verbal strokes, positive strokes like praise or appreciation, and negative strokes like put-downs. Exchange of strokes is one of the most important things that people do in their daily lives.

GAMES

A game is a recurring series of covert transactions with a beginning, middle, an end, and a payoff. The payoff (in the form of strokes) is a hidden advantage that motivates the players to participate. *The essential aspect of any game is that they are covert exchanges of strokes.*

Eric Berne, in his book "Games People Play," assigned engaging names such as "Now I've got you" "Kick me" "Why Don't You - Yes But" and "I am only trying to help" for different games. Many of these are played during doctor patient dyads. For example, when an obese diabetic plays "*Why Don't You, Yes But*" game, she asks for advice from a doctor but rejects every suggestion so that the doctor ends up exasperated.

The dyad may go on like this:

"Why don't you do exercise?" "Yes doctor, but how can I do it with my bulk?"

"Why don't you go on a strict diet?" "Yes doctor, but I get hypoglycemic symptoms if I reduce my intake."

"Why don't you then eat more of greens?" "Yes doctor, but if eat greens, I get flatulence."

And so on until the doctor gives up in exasperation (the pay-off). This type of conversation occurs repeatedly with different doctors and every exasperated doctor is one more feather in her cap. The overt level seems to be an Adult-to-Adult conversation. At a covert level, the patient's Child gets strokes when the doctor gives up and thereby "permits" her to be obese, to eat what she wants and not do any exercise.

Like every game, the above game also pays off at three different levels:

1. The biological pay-off of a game is stroke. Although, games end badly, all the players get a considerable number of strokes, both positive ("permission") and negative ("pity me") out of playing them.
2. The social pay-off of a game is time structuring. People are able to fill time -in their dull and depressing life- with an exciting activity ("I got the doctor on the defensive! He also can't help me.")
3. The existential pay-off of a game is the way in which the game confirms the existential position of each player ("Nothing ever works out for me. I shall continue to be an obese diabetic.").

Degrees

Games can be played in a range of degrees. For instance, the above example of the game is the soft (first-degree) version of the game because it is relatively harmless. The hard (third-degree) version of this game might be played by a drug addict or an alcoholic who "Yes, buts" every suggestion until his dying moment. Third degree games involve damage to health or even death.

The Existential Position

People define for themselves, early in life, what the meaning of their life or existence is. Some people decide they are OK ("Winners") and are going to have a good life; some others decide they are not OK ("losers") and will fail in some way. That is their existential position. People can feel *OK* or *not OK* about themselves and others. So there are four main existential positions:

i. "I'm OK, you're OK,"
ii. "I'm OK you're not OK,"
iii. "I'm not OK you're OK" and
iv. "I'm not OK you're not OK."

For instance, in the game of "Why Don't You, Yes But" the patient's existential position is that "nothing ever works out for me" so that every time the game is played it reinforces that position and justifies further depression.

Games are always played with responsibility and interest by everyone involved in them. In order to maintain her existential position, the patient will find doctors who will play the game with her. When they participate in the game, the doctors too believe it will end in failure. They may not be surprised when the patient rejects all advice.

SCRIPTS

People, early in their lives (during childhood) conclude that their lives will unfold in a predictable way: Short or long, healthy or unhealthy, happy or unhappy, sad or angry, successful or failure, and active or passive. This is seen as a life script. One's life script guides one's existential position.

Even when life is guided by a script, at times the person appears to evade his/her unhappy fate. This seemingly normal period of the script is called the counter-script. The counter-script is active when the person's unhappy life plan gives way to a happier period. An example is a script-driven alcoholic (or a chain smoker) gives up drinking (or smoking) transiently after his marriage. This is, however, only temporary and invariably collapses, giving way to the original script.

Perceptive doctors may see scripts and counter-scripts operate in chronic diseases. If the script is that of a "loser," it may be impossible for us to plan a sustainable treatment plan for the patient. She/he may need the help of a counselor to discard the script and begin to pursue an autonomous life-course or as Berne put it: "Close down the dismal show and put a new one on the road".

PERMISSION, PROTECTION AND POTENCY

Permission is a very important part of a transactional analysis. It happens when the counselor tells the counseled, "You can do what your parents or other people told was wrong." For example, to a teenage boy with sexual neurosis, the counsellor may say, "It is OK to masturbate and release your sexual tension; if is not bad as your parents made you believe."

When such a person takes *permission* to go against parental (and social) demands, his/her Child is apt to get very frightened. That is why *protection* is a very important part of change. Protection is given by the counselor, preferably with a group's support, to a person who is ready to change his/her script. They use nurturing parent to offer protection to the person and they say, "Don't worry, everything's going to be all right. We will take care of you, whenever you are scared." Permission and protection increase the *therapeutic potency* of a transactional analysis.

TRANSACTIONAL ANALYSIS AS A COMMUNICATION SKILL

TA can help us:

- To identify our ego states, evaluate and improve the ways in which our ego states function.
- To recognize the inner dialogs between a patient's ego states, especially those that involve a harsh demeaning critical parent pushing the person to self-destruction.
- To recognize the games that patients may play and to help them stop playing games. Giving up playing games is the first step in eventually achieving direct and honest interactions.

SUMMARY

By making clear, goal oriented therapeutic contracts, effectively analyzing patient's transactions, giving them permission to change and protecting them from their fears, it is possible for everyone to have a chance to become a happy, loving and productive person. This approach may be important in managing patients with chronic diseases like asthma and chronic pain syndrome, who have dysfunctional life.

BIBLIOGRAPHY

1. A Compilation of Core Concepts. Compiled by the ITAA Development Committee Task Force on Transactional Analysis Core Concepts Claude Steiner, Chair. August 1999. http://www.itaa-net.org/ (accessed on 19-01-2001).
2. Berne, Eric. What Do You Say After You Say Hello? New York, Grove Press, 1972.
3. Berne, Eric Games People Play. New York, Grove Press, 1964.
4. Claude Steiner http://www.itaa-net.org/ (accessed on 19-01-2001).
5. Cotterill JA. Dermatological games. British Journal of Dermatology. 105(3):31120, 1981 Sep.

PRACTICAL EXERCISES

1. Trigger video of role-play followed by discussion and clarification by the tutor. Many of the 'sitcoms' (comedy serials in TV) can be used as triggers. Discussions on the nature of transactions, the ego states in use, the existential position and life-scripts can be held.
2. Case studies of patients with chronic diseases who play "Games" and of those, who demonstrate self destructive "Life scripts." A clinical psychologist may be co-opted to conduct the plenary discussion.

ANNEXURE

2 Multidimensional Model of Healthcare

The information loaded medicine or 'info-medicine' as it is called, is often based on biomedical model and simplistic in approach. A causative agent or factor produces disease in person who consults a doctor. With the help of clinical and laboratory medicine, the disease is diagnosed and therapy is advised to control or cure of the disease. This works well on paper and in textbooks. But in real life two-thirds of cases, seen in general practice, have symptoms that do not fit into any of the diagnostic label of the biomedical model.

During the past two decades, concerned physicians around the globe have realized this anomaly. Many models and new paradigms of biopsychosocial models have been proposed. We use a multidimensional model of healthcare **(Fig. A2.1)** that perhaps represents a holistic approach to healthcare in the context of a teaching hospital.

There are four 'icebergs' (or pyramids, if you like) and two circles linking these four icebergs. The patient is at the apex and is part of a family, which is part of a community. The patient carries the knowledge, attitude and practices of the family and the community. She/he is influenced by the literary, social, cultural and economic status of self and the family. These factors, hidden in most clinical dyads, have to be considered to gain insight into the patient's mind and her/his decisions.

Similarly, the 'disease iceberg' has the following components—the illness (what the patient perceives), the disease (what the doctor perceives), the internal environment, causative agent/factor, and finally, the external environment and aggravating or triggering factors. The basic needs of a human being, viz. food, water, clothes, shelter and energy form a part of this.

The third 'iceberg' has doctor who is the most visible to the patients. He is supported by healthcare team and diagnostic facility. Healthcare system—primary, secondary and tertiary care—functioning at the locality and the country are at the bottom. Alternative systems of medicine form another face of the iceberg. Availability, appropriateness, acceptability, affordability, accessibility are major concerns here.

The fourth is the 'treatment iceberg.' Its visible part is the drug and non-drug therapy advised by the doctor. Availability, accessibility, acceptability and affordability of these therapies form its mid-portion. Production and procurement at a macrolevel forms the bottom of this iceberg. Current furore on highly active antiretroviral therapy (HAART) in the third world is an excellent example of these aspects of healthcare.

Finally, transport, communication and internet link these four elements. Media form part of the communication. These are in the outer circle. Activists and professional organizations can act upon and influence healthcare delivery while the governments can regulate as well as act decisively on any of these. Inner circle represent them.

This model may sound complicated enough to be an acceptable paradigm of holistic healthcare. However, is it useful especially to a teaching hospital? My experience with interns has been quite revealing. Let us see two examples discussed by the medicos:

1. Rasheed, a diabetic patient was a difficult case to control. He was on tablets and insulin injections. His family doctor repeatedly referred him for better control. When an intern interviewed him regarding sociocultural acceptance of therapy, he discovered that, Rasheed never took the injections for he believed that the insulin was derived from pork. His religion proscribed pork. He was reluctant to disclose this on his own for fear of ridicule.
2. A 15-year-old boy had fever for 2 months. He had disseminated tuberculosis. In spite of his family having had two cases of lung TB, none of them suspected TB in this boy "because he had no cough or blood spitting". On review, the intern found that none of the campaigns on TB stress on extrapulmonary TB. Hence, the community is generally unaware of other forms of TB resulting in serious delay in seeking treatment.

After using the model in several clinical dyads, the interns opined, "*The conventional history elicitation covers many personal and family details. The use of the healthcare model added newer dimensions in understanding a case, especially a chronic one. It also helped us to offer meaningful advice to such cases.*"

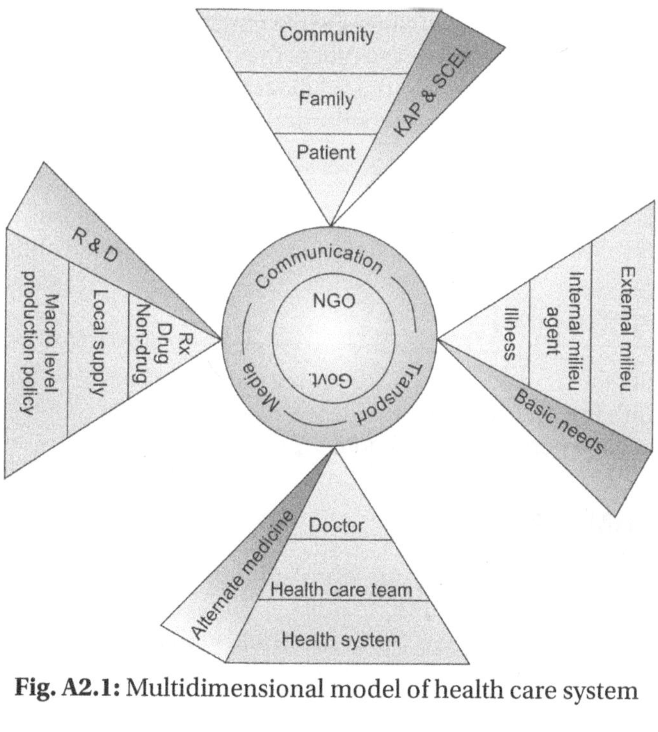

Fig. A2.1: Multidimensional model of health care system

Abbreviation

KAP - Knowledge, Attitude & Practice
SCEL - Social, Cultural, Economic & Literary
R & D - Research & Development
NGO - Non Government organization
Govt. - Government

Sources: Sethuraman KR, A holistic perspective in Medicine. In S. Chandrasekar *et al.* Beyond Rational Therapy . EQUIP Society, P.B. No. 8., Pondicherry 1995. (Reproduced with permission from Publisher)

Annexure

3 The Kalamazoo Consensus Statement: Essential Elements of Communication in Medical Encounters

BUILD A RELATIONSHIP: THE FUNDAMENTAL COMMUNICATION TASK

A strong, therapeutic, and effective relationship is the sine qua non of physician–patient communication. The group endorses a patient-centered, or relationship-centered, approach to care, which emphasizes both the patient's disease and his or her illness experience. This requires eliciting the patient's story of illness while guiding the interview through a process of diagnostic reasoning. It also requires awareness that the ideas, feelings, and values of both the patient and the physician influence the relationship. Further, this approach regards the physician–patient relationship as a partnership, and respects patients' active participation in decision making.

The task of building a relationship is also relevant for work with patients' families and support networks. In essence, building a relationship is an ongoing task within and across encounters: it subsumes the more sequentially ordered sets of tasks identified below.

OPEN THE DISCUSSION

- Allow the patient to complete his or her opening statement
- Elicit the patient's full set of concerns
- Establish/maintain a personal connection.

GATHER INFORMATION

- Use open-ended and closed-ended questions appropriately
- Structure, clarify, and summarize information
- Actively listen using nonverbal (e.g. eye contact) and verbal (e.g. words of encouragement) techniques.

UNDERSTAND THE PATIENT'S PERSPECTIVE

- Explore contextual factors (e.g. family, culture, gender, age, socioeconomic status and spirituality)
- Explore beliefs, concerns, and expectations about health and illness
- Acknowledge and respond to the patient's ideas, feelings and values.

SHARE INFORMATION

- Use language which patient can understand
- Check for understanding
- Encourage questions.

REACH AGREEMENT ON PROBLEMS AND PLANS

- Encourage the patient to participate in decisions to the extent he or she desires
- Check the patient's willingness and ability to follow the plan
- Identify and enlist resources and supports.

PROVIDE CLOSURE

- Ask whether the patient has other issues or concerns
- Summarize and affirm agreement with the plan of action
- Discuss follow-up (e.g. next visit, plan for unexpected outcomes)

Reference: *Acad. Med.* ,2001;76:390-393. *available at http://journals.lww.com/academicmedicine/toc/2001/04000*

ANNEXURE

4

Roter Interaction Analysis System (RIAS)

The RIAS was devised by Debra Roter in the late 1970's. Over 30 years of development has given it a high standard of reliability and validity. The RIAS is currently the most widely used method of coding medical interactions (URL: http://riasworks.com/resources.html).

RIAS CODING CATEGORIES

- Personal remarks, social conversation
- Laughs, tells jokes
- Shows concern or worry
- Reassures, encourages or show optimism
- Shows approval—direct
- Gives compliment—general
- Shows disapproval—direct
- Shows criticism—general
- Shows agreement or understanding
- Back-channel responses (physician only)
- Empathy statements
- Legitimizing statements
- Partnership statements (physician only)
- Self-disclosure statements (physician only)
- Asks for reassurance
- Transition words
- Gives orientation, instructions
- Paraphrase/checks for understanding
- Asks for understanding
- Bid for repetition
- Asks for opinion (physician only)
- Asks for permission (physician only)
- Asks closed-ended questions—medical condition
- Asks closed-ended questions—therapeutic regimen
- Asks closed-ended questions—lifestyle

- Asks closed-ended questions—psychosocial
- Asks closed-ended questions—other
- Asks open-ended questions—medical condition
- Asks open-ended questions-therapeutic regimen
- Asks open-ended questions—lifestyle
- Asks open-ended questions—psychosocial
- Asks open-ended questions—other
- Gives information—medical condition
- Gives information—therapeutic regimen
- Gives information—lifestyle
- Gives information—psychosocial
- Gives information—other
- Counsels—medical condition/therapeutic regimen (physician only)
- Counsels—lifestyle/psychosocial (physician only)
- Requests for services (patient only)
- Unintelligible utterances.

GLOBAL AFFECT RATINGS

In addition to utterance by utterance categorization, the affect or emotional context of the dialog is rated as well. These ratings are based on overall affective impressions of the speakers on such dimensions as dominance, assertiveness, friendliness, warmth, attentiveness, and respectfulness.

Index

A

B

C

N

O

P

Q

R

S

T

V

W